OXFORD PAIN MANAGEMENT LIBRARY

Neuropathic Pain

Second Edition

OXFORD PAIN MANAGEMENT LIBRARY

Neuropathic Pain

Second Edition

Editor

Dr Michael I. Bennett
Professor of Palliative Medicine
School of Health and Medicine
Lancaster University
Lancaster
LA1 4YT

OXFORD
UNIVERSITY PRESS

OXFORD
UNIVERSITY PRESS

Great Clarendon Street, Oxford OX2 6DP

Oxford University Press is a department of the University of Oxford.
It furthers the University's objective of excellence in research, scholarship,
and education by publishing worldwide in

Oxford New York

Auckland Cape Town Dar es Salaam Hong Kong Karachi
Kuala Lumpur Madrid Melbourne Mexico City Nairobi
New Delhi Shanghai Taipei Toronto

With offices in

Argentina Austria Brazil Chile Czech Republic France Greece
Guatemala Hungary Italy Japan Poland Portugal Singapore
South Korea Switzerland Thailand Turkey Ukraine Vietnam

Oxford is a registered trade mark of Oxford University Press
in the UK and in certain other countries

Published in the United States
by Oxford University Press Inc., New York

First published 2006
Second edition published 2010

British Library Cataloguing in Publication Data
Data available

Library of Congress Cataloging in Publication Data
Data available

Typeset by Newgen Imaging Systems (P) Ltd., Chennai, India
Printed in Great Britain
on acid-free paper by
Ashford Colour Press Ltd., Gosport, Hampshire
ISBN 978–0–19–956367–8

10 9 8 7 6 5 4 3 2 1

Contents

Contributors

Michael I. Bennett

Professor of Palliative Medicine
School of Health and Medicine
Lancaster University
Lancaster
LA1 4YT

David Bowsher

Emeritus Hon. Consultant
Neurologist (Pain Relief)
Former Reader in Neurological
Sciences, University of Liverpool
Pain Relief Foundation
Clinical Sciences Centre
University Hospital Aintree
Lower lane
Liverpool
L9 7AL

Dudley Bush

Consultant Anaesthetist
Pain Management Service
L Ward
Seacroft Hospital
York Road
Leeds
LS14 6UH

S. José Closs

Professor of Nursing Research
School of Healthcare
Baines Wing
University of Leeds
Leeds
LS2 9UT

Marie Fallon

Professor of Palliative Medicine
University of Edinburgh
Edinburgh Cancer Centre
Western General Hospital
Crewe Road
Edinburgh
EH4 2XU

Cameron Fergus

Specialist Registrar in Palliative
Medicine
Edinburgh Cancer Centre
Western General Hospital
Crewe Road
Edinburgh
EH4 2XU

Rainer Freynhagen

Associate Professor, Head
Department of Anaesthesiology,
Critical Care Medicine,
Pain Therapy & Palliative Care,
Pain Center Lake Starnberg,
Benedictus Krankenhaus
Tutzing, 82327
Germany

Irene J. Higginson

Professor of Palliative Care
Department of Palliative Care
Policy and Rehabilitation
Weston Education Centre
King's College London

Mark I. Johnson

Professor of Pain and Analgesia
Faculty of Health
Leeds Metropolitan University
Calverley Street
Leeds
LS1 3HE

Iain Jones

Consultant in Anaesthesia and
Pain Management
Royal Victoria Infirmary
Queen Victoria Road
Newcastle upon Tyne
NE1 4NP

Barry J.A. Laird

Research Fellow in Palliative
Medicine
University of Edinburgh
Edinburgh Cancer Research
Centre
Western General Hospital
Edinburgh

Gary McCleane

Consultant in Pain Management
Rampark Pain Centre
2 Rampark
Dromore Road
Lurgan
N. Ireland
BT66 7JH

Henry J. McQuay

Nuffield Professor of Clinical
Anaesthetics
University of Oxford
Nuffied Department of
Anaesthetics
John Radcliffe Hospital
Oxford
OX3 9D4

Fliss E. Murtagh

Clinical Senior Lecturer in
Palliative Medicine
Department of Palliative Care
Policy and Rehabilitation
Weston Education Centre
King's College
London

Tim Nash

Honorary Senior Lecturer
Department of Neuroscience
University of Liverpool
Consultant in Pain Medicine
Walton Centre for Neurology
and Neurosurgery
Lower Lane
Fazakerley
Liverpool
L9 7LJ

Roman Rolke

Department of Neurology
University Medical Center
Johannes Gutenberg-University
Langenbeckstr. 1
55131 Mainz
Germany

Brian A. Simpson

Consultant Neurosurgeon
Department of Neurosurgery
University Hospital of Wales
Heath Park
Cardiff
CF14 4XW

Karen H. Simpson

Consultant in Pain
Management and Senior
Clincal Lecturer
Leeds Teaching Hospitals Trust
Seacroft Hospital
York Road
Leeds
LS14 6UH

Blair H. Smith

Professor of Primary Care
Medicine
Head of Section
General Practice and
Community Medical Education
University of Aberdeen
Foresterhill Health Centre
Westburn Road
Aberdeen
AB25 2AY

Nicola Torrance

Research Fellow
Department of General
Practice and Primary Care
University of Aberdeen
Fosterhill Health Centre
Westburn Road
Aberdeen
AB25 2AY

Catherine E. Urch
Honorary Senior Lecturer
UCL and Imperial College
Consultant in Palliative Medicine
St Mary's and Royal Brompton
Hospitals
Department of Palliative Care
St Mary's Hospital
Praed Street
Paddington
W2 1NY

Philip Wiffen
Co-ordinating Editor
Cochrane Pain & Palliative
Care Group
Pain Relief Unit
Churchill Hospital
Oxford
OX3 7LJ

Preface

Since the first edition of this book was published in 2006, research in neuropathic pain has progressed and continues to impact on clinical practice. This second edition of Oxford Pain Management Library book *Neuropathic Pain* reflects these developments in significant updates to existing chapters and also the addition of new chapters which cover neuropathic back pain and a more detailed chapter on clinical assessment.

The aim of the book remains that of being a concise companion for health care professionals across the range of primary care, and medical and surgical specialties. Neuropathic pain continues to be a chronic condition that can blight people's lives. While we all hope that research can deliver better treatments, implementing existing knowledge on assessment and diagnosis and ensuring prompt treatment with current therapies, can still go a long way to improving the quality of life for many. I hope that this book can help in that endeavour.

Michael Bennett
Lancaster, September 2009

Abbreviations

AL-TENS	acupuncture-like TENS
ASIC	acid-sensing receptors
ATP	adenosine tri-phosphate
CCK	cholecystokinin
CI	confidence intervals
CNP	central neuropathic pain
CPB	coeliac plexus block
CPSMV	Chronic Pain associated with various combinations of positive and negative Sensory, Motor and Vasomotor phenomena
CPSP	central post-stroke pain
CRPS	complex regional pain syndrome
DMA	dynamic mechanical allodynia
DN4	Douleur Neuropathique 4
DRG	dorsal root ganglion
EFNS	European Federation of Neurological Societies
fMRI	functional magnetic resonance imaging
GABA	gamma amino butyric acid
GPs	general practitioners
HIV	human immunodeficiency virus
HSAN	hereditary sensory and autonomic neuropathy
IASP	International Association for the Study of Pain
ICVDD	intracerebroventricular drug delivery
IPG	implanted pulse generator
IT	intrathecal
ITDD	intrathecal drug delivery
IV	intravenous
LANSS	Leeds Assessment of Neuropathic Symptoms and Signs
LBP	low back pain
LEP	laser-evoked potentials
MEG	magneto-encephalography
MRI	magnetic resonance imaging
NMDA	N-methyl D-aspartate receptor

NNH	needed to harm
NNT	number-needed-to-treat
NOP	nociceptin orphanin FQ peptide
NPQ	Neuropathic Pain Questionnaire
NPS	Neuropathic Pain Scale
NPSI	Neuropathic Pain Symptom Inventory
NSPB	neurolytic sympathetic plexus blocks
PAG	peri-aquaductal grey
PDN	painful diabetic neuropathy
PET	positron emission tomography
PHN	postherpetic neuralgia
QST	quantitative sensory testing
RCTs	randomized controlled trials
RF	radiofrequency
RSD	reflex sympathetic dystrophy
RVM	rostro-ventral medulla
SCI	spinal cord injury
SCS	spinal cord stimulation
SEP	somatosensory-evoked potentials
SHPB	superior hypogastric plexus block
SIP	sympathetically independent pain
S–LANSS	Leeds Assessment of Neuropathic Symptoms and Signs
SMP	sympathetically maintained pain
SNRIs	serotonin noradrenaline re-uptake inhibitors
SNS	sympathetic nervous system
SSRIs	selective serotonin re-uptake inhibitors
STRICTA	STandards for Reporting Interventions in Controlled Trails of Acupuncture
TCAs	tricyclic antidepressants
TENS	transcutaneous electrical nerve stimulation
VDCC	voltage-dependent calcium channels

Chapter 1

Theories, history, and current taxonomy

Michael I. Bennett

Key points

- Pain is a complex experience of somatic mechanisms and psychological influences (affective and cognitive) and, as such, is always subjective in nature
- The nervous system is capable of substantial plasticity; it can change structure and function in response to development, injury, or experience
- Nociceptive or inflammatory pain arises from normal activation of pain pathways
- Neuropathic pain is pain arising as a direct consequence of a lesion or disease affecting the somatosensory system (abnormal activation of pain pathways)
- Pain is usually classified by mechanism (nociceptive or neuropathic), context (physiological or pathological), and location (somatic, visceral, etc.).

1.1 Theories of pain

1.1.1 Pre-renaissance

Theories of pain date to ancient civilizations where pain was thought to be inflicted by gods or due to imbalances in 'vital energies' or 'body humours'. At this time, Aristotle proposed that the heart was the centre of sensation, and thus pain was an affective quality. Hippocrates, however, viewed the brain as the centre of sensation. Some 2,000 years later, Descartes in the early seventeenth century described nerves as tubes containing threads, each connecting an area of skin directly to the brain, the seat of sensation. These threads transmitted signals in a 'hard-wired' fashion.

1.1.2 Early science

By the late nineteenth century, two distinct pain theories had emerged. The first proposed that pain is a specific sensation served by dedicated nerves independent of other sensations. This subsequently became known as the 'specificity theory'. A second pain theory, the 'summation theory', was proposed shortly after which suggested that pain was the product of any sensory modality given a stimulus of sufficient intensity. The earlier view of pain as an affective quality remained until a new theory of pain emerged in the 1950s. This 'sensory interaction theory' incorporated two components: the sensation of pain (dependent on physiological processes) and the reaction to it (dependent on cognitive and affective processes). This theory proposed the involvement of two systems in pain transmission. One consisted of slowly conducting small fibres whose activation produced painful sensations. The other consisted of faster-conducting larger fibres whose activation inhibited transmission of small fibre impulses in the dorsal horn.

1.1.3 Gate-control theory

The gate-control theory was effectively a synthesis of the strongest elements of all these main theories. It recognized the specificity of peripheral pain systems, central summation, and input modulation via larger sensory fibres and psychological influences. The gate-control theory proposed a spinal gating mechanism in the dorsal horn that was influenced by the relative amounts of activity in large and small fibres and by descending controls from the brain. Thus, pain is a complex experience of somatic mechanisms and psychological influences (affective and cognitive) and, as such, is always subjective in nature.

1.1.4 Current model

Increasing neuroscience evidence suggests that the nervous system is capable of substantial plasticity. This is the ordered alteration of structure or function due to development, experience, or injury. Central neurons have the capacity to change their responsiveness in spatial, temporal, and amplitude aspects to a given stimulus, especially if the stimulus is chronic. This 'jungle of neurochemical anatomy' can undoubtedly account for this plastic nature but the exact mechanisms are still being elucidated. The plasticity theory is the most comprehensive pain model to date.

1.2 Classification of pain

1.2.1 Physiological or pathological?

Attempts at the classification of pain continue to evolve but, to date, all generally reflect the underlying pathophysiological mechanisms that are thought to *initiate* the pain. Although this classification of pain is simplistic, it affords a working paradigm in the pain clinic and is generally accepted by practitioners.

Pain classifications generally propose that pain is either physiological (normal) or pathological (abnormal), although there is no universally accepted system. Physiological pain results from the activation of peripheral nociceptive afferents by noxious (potentially harmful) stimuli assuming baseline sensitivity of the sensory system and serves to warn of impending tissue injury. Here, pain is a normal experience that is essential to the survival of the individual though a well argued editorial suggests that this concept may be flawed (see Nash 2005).

Pathological pain is distinguished by a change in baseline sensitivity of the nervous system and occurs after injury. This serves to protect the individual from further injury while healing occurs, an adaptive response. Pathological pain is termed 'maladaptive' when the sensitivity of the sensory system does not return to normal after tissue healing. Nociceptive pain is pain that occurs due to normal activation of the nociceptive system either by impending tissue injury or ongoing tissue destruction or inflammation.

This model has been developed further into a three-level classification which incorporates firstly the mechanism (nociceptive or neuropathic), then the context (physiological or pathological), and finally the location (somatic, e.g. bone; or visceral, e.g. bowel) (Figure 1.1).

1.2.2 Mechanism based

Recently, a more fundamental mechanism-based classification of pain has been proposed. In this system, pain symptoms, mechanisms, and syndromes form a new hierarchy which does not involve traditional dichotomies such as malignant/non-malignant or acute/chronic. Two broad pain categories are identified—tissue injury pain (inflammatory) or nervous system injury pain—both of which encompass a number of universal mechanisms.

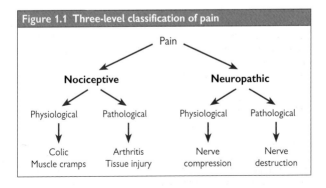

Figure 1.1 Three-level classification of pain

Pain

Nociceptive   Neuropathic

Physiological   Pathological   Physiological   Pathological

Colic   Arthritis   Nerve   Nerve
Muscle cramps   Tissue injury   compression   destruction

1.3 **History of neuropathic pain**

Dysfunction of the nervous system as a cause of chronic pain had been recognized by Galen in the second century AD, but it was after the Middle Ages that more consistent reports have been found. The increasing use of guns in wars from the seventeenth century onwards accounted for a great deal of traumatic nerve injury suffered by those that survived such injuries. Another feature of military life that began around this time was the recording and treatment of injuries by medical and nursing personnel accompanying the army.

Several of these accounts match contemporary descriptions of neuropathic pain. Dr Weir-Mitchell famously published his descriptions of pain associated with peripheral nerve injuries in Unionist soldiers of the American Civil War in 1864 and coined the term 'causalgia'. Ideas as to the mechanisms of pain that resulted from neural injury surfaced early in the twentieth century. However, steady growth of neuropathic pain research did not occur until the late 1970s when the special nature of neuropathic pain had been recognized and distinct terminology had emerged.

1.4 **Current taxonomy**

1.4.1 **Neuropathic pain definitions**

Neuropathy is defined as the disturbance of function or pathological change in a nerve. Since 1994, the definition for neuropathic pain by the International Association for the Study of Pain (IASP) has been 'pain initiated or caused by a primary lesion or dysfunction of the nervous system'. However, in 2008 IASP approved a change of definition to 'pain arising as a direct consequence of a lesion or disease affecting the somatosensory system'. This effectively means that dysfunction without evidence of injury is no longer regarded as meeting the criteria for neuropathic pain.

Neuropathic pain is best thought of as an *abnormal* activation of pain pathways and can occur as a result of injury to peripheral nerves and posterior roots (peripheral neuropathic pain) and spinal cord and brain (central pain). Table 1.1 contains examples of clinical neuropathic pains.

Despite 'neuropathic pain' being the preferred term, there has been some confusion over the terminology of this pain-generating mechanism. Some authors prefer the term 'neurogenic pain' while others prefer 'deafferentation pain' (this denotes complete nerve destruction with loss of afferent input beyond this point). Both are used as umbrella terms for peripheral neuropathic pain and central neuropathic pain.

Table 1.1 Examples of neuropathic pain		
Origin of pain	Structure	Example
Peripheral nervous system	Nerve	Neuroma
		Diabetic neuropathy
		Phantom limb pain
		Trigeminal neuralgia
		Lumbosacral plexopathy
	Dorsal root	Post-herpetic neuralgia
		Brachial plexus avulsion
Central nervous system	Spinal cord	Spinal cord injury
		Spinal cord ischaemia
	Brain	Wallenberg's syndrome
		Multiple sclerosis

1.4.2 Types of neuropathic pain

The distinction between physiological and pathological neuropathic pain has been made. The former includes nerve compression pain which produces a *reversible* dysfunction of the nerve provided the compression is transient. Clinically, the symptoms of nerve compression are not easy to distinguish from nerve destruction.

1.4.3 Role of autonomic system

Until recently, pain associated with autonomic dysfunction was considered separately from neuropathic pain. It remains a controversial area particularly with the recent redefinition of neuropathic pain. Some pains with autonomic dysfunction do not have clear nerve damage even though the clinical features are similar to those of other neuropathic pains. However, autonomic dysfunction in association with demonstrable nerve injury is clearly recognized as neuropathic pain.

Confusion over the classification of autonomic dysfunction remains. Some authors divide pain associated with autonomic dysfunction into sympathetically maintained pain (SMP) or sympathetically independent pain (SIP) according to whether the patient's pain improves or not after sympathetic blockade, though this has been shown to be an unreliable test.

Sympathetic pain has undergone several redefinitions including CPSMV (Chronic Pain associated with various combinations of positive and negative Sensory, Motor and Vasomotor phenomena). In the last 10 years it has come to be known as Complex Regional Pain Syndrome (see Chapter 8). The change in definition reflects the unpredictable contribution of autonomic dysfunction to neuropathic pain and the uncertainty over causal mechanisms.

1.5 Can pain be more or less neuropathic?

When assessing a patient with chronic pain, it is tempting to think that their underlying pain mechanism is either nociceptive or neuropathic, and current taxonomy encourages this view. However, experienced clinicians know that this is an oversimplification. In reality, patients present with a variety of clinical features, including anatomical and physiological abnormalities, which form a very mixed picture.

An emerging view is that pain, and chronic pain in particular, can be more or less neuropathic. In other words, the features of chronic pain experienced by any patient reflect the balance between underlying nociceptive and neuropathic mechanisms.

This viewpoint is supported by the recent IASP taxonomy which proposes that neuropathic pain be graded as definite, probable and possible. These categories are empirical and the suggested criteria for each have yet to be validated. Interestingly, research using screening tools for neuropathic pain (see Chapter 5) reveals a spectrum of patient responses in patients with chronic pain. This spectrum correlates well with responses by clinicians when asked 'what is the certainty that neuropathic pain exists in this patient?' This evidence underlies the concept that there is considerable variance in the clinical expression of neuropathic mechanisms.

From a diagnostic perspective, the question for clinicians is not 'is this pain neuropathic or nociceptive?' but 'what is the probability that neuropathic mechanisms are responsible for this chronic pain state?' (not at all, possibly, probably or definitely). Although this view offers a more flexible clinical model and therefore opens up treatment opportunities, it requires further validation and testing.

Key references

Attal, N. and Bouhassira, D. (2004). Can pain be more or less neuropathic? *Pain*, **110**, 510–11.

Backonja, M.M. (2003). Defining neuropathic pain. *Anesth. Analg.*, **97**, 785–90.

Bennett, M.I., Smith, B.H., Torrance, N., Lee, A.J. (2006). Can pain be more or less neuropathic? Comparison of symptom assessment tools with ratings of certainty by clinicians. *Pain*, **122**(3), 289–94.

Bennett, G.J. (2003). Neuropathic pain: a crisis of definition? *Anesth. Analg.*, **97**, 619–20.

Melzack, R. and Wall, P.D. (1965). Pain mechanisms: a new theory. *Science*, **150**, 971–9.

Merskey, H. and Bogduk, N. (1994). *Classification of chronic pain: descriptions of chronic pain syndromes and definitions of pain terms* (2nd edn). IASP Press, Seattle.

Nash, T. (2005). 'What use is pain?' *British Journal of Anaesthesia*, **94**(2), 146–9.

Treede R.D., Jensen T.S., Campbell J.N., Cruccu G., Dostrovsky J.O., Griffin J.W., *et al.* (2008). Neuropathic pain: redefinition and a grading system for clinical and research purposes. *Neurology*, **70**(18), 1630–5.

Woolf, C.J., Bennett, G.J., Doherty, M., Dubner, R., Kidd, B., Koltzenburg, M., et al. (1998). Towards a mechanism-based classification of pain? *Pain*, **77**, 227–9.

Chapter 2

Pathophysiology of neuropathic pain

Catherine E. Urch

> **Key points**
>
> - Noxious stimuli are coded and transmitted via A and C primary afferent neurons in the periphery to the dorsal horn of the spinal cord
> - In the dorsal horn, transmission of noxious stimuli involves the neurotransmitters glutamate and substance P, but input can be inhibited or amplified by other influences
> - Damage to peripheral nerves can result in reduced firing thresholds, ectopic discharges, and cross-talk (activation of adjacent normal nerves)
> - Abnormal peripheral input or direct damage to the central nervous system leads to hyperexcitability and loss of inhibition
> - Neuropathic pain states can impact on control of descending inhibitory pathways from higher brain centres.

Pain arising after nerve injury or damage is a challenge to both clinicians and scientists. In other areas of nerve damage, sensory loss is expected, such as with vision. However, the question is when neuronal damage is inflicted on nociceptive neurons, why is there both loss, in the form of numbness, and abnormal gains in the form of pain and hyperalgesia?

2.1 Normal transmission

2.1.1 Activation in the periphery

Pain is normally elicited only when a noxious (potentially harmful) stimulus activates the high-threshold peripheral nociceptors. The peripheral nervous system is differentiated into Aβ fibres, which are activated by non-noxious (non-harmful) stimuli; and Aδ and C primary afferent fibres, which specifically code for noxious stimuli, such as heat, chemical, pressure, and inflammation. These stimuli activate specific receptors on the neuron (such as acid-sensing receptors [ASIC] and prostaglandin receptors), which in turn allow the neuron to depolarize by an influx of positive ions, usually sodium and calcium. Once a threshold is reached the neuron continues to carry the depolarization up to its cell body, the dorsal root ganglion (DRG), and the dorsal horn within the spinal cord.

2.1.2 Activity in the central nervous system

Once in the spinal cord the neuron releases transmitters, such as glutamate and substance P, which travel across the synapse to the post-synaptic neurons and glial cells. The neurons can be inhibitory (gamma amino butyric acid [GABA]-ergic) or excitatory interneurons, whilst the glial cells play an active role in removing and releasing neurotransmitters. The dorsal horn can modulate the input of the primary afferent neuron to allow magnification (excitation, with 'wind-up') or reduction (inhibition). The net result is passed via the ascending tracts (such as spinothalamic, parabrachial) to the higher brain centres involved in the coding, modulating, and the experience of pain. The brain in turn sends excitatory and inhibitory signals back to the dorsal horn via the descending pathways, which in turn further modulate the output.

2.2 Peripheral changes following damage

Neuropathic pain is characterized by spontaneous pain (stimulus-independent), hyperalgesia (increased pain to a given noxious stimulus), and allodynia (pain arising from non-noxious stimuli). Some of these clinical characteristics may be explained by the alterations that occur within the peripheral nerves following damage.

2.2.1 Reduced thresholds

If the milieu surrounding a peripheral neuron is altered, or the nerve is compressed or damaged, the receptors that normally transduce stimuli at certain intensities can be activated at lower intensities. For example, with cell damage, death, or inflammation, the pH can be reduced and thus activate the ASIC channels, or Adenosine Tri-Phosphate (ATP) receptors (P_2X_3). This in turn can lead to the neuron being always partially or totally depolarized. In the former, it wouldn't take much further activation, say by a prostaglandin or bradykinin receptor activation, to make the neuron fire. The normally high-threshold neuron will now be activated with a lower threshold stimulus, which is seen in hyperalgesia.

2.2.2 Altered transmission

Normal transmission relies on ordered sequential functioning of sodium and calcium channels, allowing depolarization to occur in a specific place and time. In damaged neurons, perhaps caused by transection following surgery or amputation, the severed neuron responds to the loss of its distal portion by trying to regrow ('sprouting'), forming a neuroma which is a whorl of neuronal tissue with or without myelin. Neurons also develop abnormal accumulations of sodium and calcium channels, which are not only abnormal in density (increased), but also undergo a change in character and activation properties.

There are nine different sodium channels currently identified which possess different characteristics with respect to what voltage they open at, how long they stay open, how quickly they close (inactivate), and the refractory time before reopening. The distribution of sodium channels alters with development, type of neuron, and in response to damage. For example, it has been shown that a fetal sodium channel, $Na_v1.3$, is up-regulated following neuropathy, $Na_v1.8$ is located on small-diameter primary afferents (Aδ and C fibres), whilst $Na_v1.7$ is on all size fibres. Work suggests that the differential expression and accumulation of sodium channels is responsible for spontaneous discharges in damaged neurons (called ectopic discharges), which may be perceived as spontaneous pain. Normally, nerve impulses are generated at sensory terminals. In pathological states, impulses may arise from the damaged part of the axon, or from abnormal accumulations of sodium channels on neighbouring non-damged axons, and propagate toward both the central nervous system and the periphery. Such ectopic discharges may also arise from local patches of demyelination, neuroma, and the dorsal root ganglion.

Likewise, the calcium channels belong to a large family, and are differentially located depending on neuronal type and damage. All calcium channels contain a sub-unit $a_2\delta$, which is an important therapeutic target for gabapentin. Remodelling of other membrane channels is important, such as potassium channels, if not as well characterized (Figure 2.1).

2.2.3 **Other peripheral changes**

The chaotic depolarization and transmission affects events:

- within the neuron—such as altered retrograde translation of nerve growth factor
- within the dorsal root ganglion—activation of *c-fos* and other genes, with the result of altered receptor and secondary messenger translation
- between neurons
- within the dorsal horn.

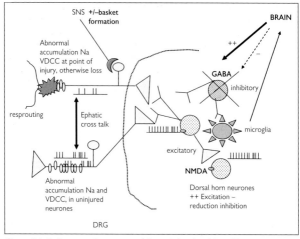

Figure 2.1 A diagrammatic summary of the peripheral and dorsal horn pro-excitatory changes following a peripheral nerve injury. In the periphery, there is an increase in density and activity of sodium (Na) and voltage-dependent calcium channels (VDCC), leading to ectopic discharge. There is also ephatic cross-talk between damaged and undamaged neurons and sprouting of the damaged neuron, all leading to an increase in receptive field size. In some cases the sympathetic nervous system (SNS) may form aberrant sprouting, leading to basket formation around abnormal dorsal root ganglion (DRG). The dorsal horn is pro-excitatory, as illustrated by an increasing number of action potentials with each inter-neuron. The excitation is in part driven by the activation of NMDA receptors, amongst others, and the overall reduction of inhibition, either intrinsic—GABA-ergic loss, inhibited opioid receptors—or extrinsic—reduced descending inhibition and increased descending facilitation.

In the periphery, the abnormal neuronal sprouting can lead to an enlargement of the receptive field (area of body) that feeds the abnormal pain transmission. These nerve endings also 'cross-talk' to other non-damaged nerves, in turn altering the normal nerves to become abnormal and chaotic. Likewise, the damaged neuron itself engages in 'ephatic' cross-talk to non-damaged neurons within its bundle. This cross-talk causes a synchronous depolarization and perpetuates the pathological characteristics onto otherwise normal non-damaged neurons (for example accumulation of sodium channels).

2.3 **Alterations within the dorsal horn**

2.3.1 **Peripheral inputs**

The dorsal horn is a central point of modulation of normal pain signals, and is also vital to the onward transmission of the abnormal and chaotic inputs from damaged (and adjacent) non-damaged neurons.

The A and C fibres terminate predominantly in the superficial layers (lamina I and II) of the dorsal horn, also A in lamina V, and the non-noxious Aβ fibres terminate in lamina III. Work of some years ago suggested that there was abnormal resprouting of A fibres into lamina II, thus allowing non-painful thresholds to be translated in the dorsal horn as pain. This would have accounted nicely for the symptom of allodynia. This theory, whilst widely quoted and beguiling in its neatness, has in many elements been disproved and dorsal horn neuronal reorganization should be viewed as contentious. It appears that C fibres take on characteristics of, and express receptors that are normally confined to, low-threshold Aβ fibres.

2.3.2 Role of NMDA receptors

Within the dorsal horn the abnormal primary afferent inputs result in areas of 'silence' (with no input) and areas of chaotic over-activity. The increased release of neurotransmitters allows the prolonged depolarization of the post-synaptic neurons, and the activation of the N-methyl D-aspartate (NMDA) receptor. This receptor is important, as it usually remains closed by magnesium ion block until both the cell is depolarized and there continues to be glutamate (and glycine) binding to the receptor (Figure 2.2; see also Chapter 13). Once these multiple events occur, the receptor opens and allows a flood of calcium and sodium into the cell. The effect is one of massive excitation within the

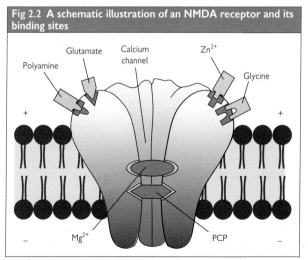

Fig 2.2 A schematic illustration of an NMDA receptor and its binding sites

Figure 2.2 reproduced with permission from Neil Camson *Foundations of Physiological Psychology*, 6e. Published by Allyn and Bacon, Boston, MA. Copyright © 2004 by Pearson Education.

neuron, known as 'wind-up', a greatly increased response to a given stimuli. Increase of calcium within the cell not only activates and depolarizes it, but also sets in train a series of events that modifies receptors (either more open or more closed), activates secondary messenger pathways, alters gene expression, increases the production of excitatory gases such as nitric oxide, and other effects. The overall effect is one of neuronal excitation.

In addition it appears that there is an overall reduction in the inhibition within the dorsal horn, either by loss or down-regulation of GABA-ergic neurons, or loss of active intrinsic opioid receptors, combined with reduction in descending inhibitory pathways (see Figure 2.1).

2.4 **Alterations centrally**

2.4.1 **Descending pathways**

Serotonergic pathways appear to be central in the descending facilitatory pathway. From lamina I of the dorsal horn, the parabrachial pathway ascends to the brainstem (hypothalamus, perception). The signals are modulated and transmitted to the peri-aquaductal grey (PAG) and rostro-ventral medulla (RVM) from where the descending system commences and terminates back within the spinal cord. It has been shown that the attention/distraction centre of the PAG is aberrant in humans with chronic pain, who could not activate descending inhibition. It must be remembered that whilst the ascending spinothalamic pathways retain a strict location mapping, the parabrachial and descending systems are diffuse and lack location map (Figure 2.3).

2.4.2 **Control of descending pathways**

The peripheral and dorsal horn alterations have been investigated extensively for decades in animal models. The areas are readily accessible and much has been elucidated about the pathophysiological state that follows neuropathic injury, which has been largely confirmed in human studies.

The more central areas within the brain have remained a black box for some time. However, over the last decade sophisticated animal work within the RVM and PAG have revealed a complex web of interconnecting neurons, with specific 'on', 'off', and 'neutral' cells which are central in controlling descending pathways back to the dorsal horn. These areas in turn have projections to and from multiple other areas such as the sensory cortex and hypothalamus. The recent refinement of functional magnetic resonance imaging (fMRI) and positron emission tomography (PET) imaging has allowed a more clinically based approach to understanding the complex interconnections and plasticity within the brain following neuropathic injury (Figure 2.3).

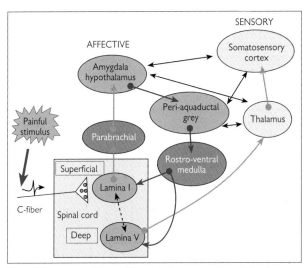

Figure 2.3 A summary of some of the interactions between the peripheral neurons, dorsal horn, and higher centres in the brain. As illustrated, the noxious coding Aδ and C fibres terminate in the superficial (lamina I /II) and deep (lamina V) dorsal horn. However, the ascending pathways are distinct. The predominant pathway to the sensory cortex, coding for intensity and location of the stimulus, is via the spinothalamic tract, whilst the parabrachial pathway is predominantely responsible for linking lamina I with the hypothalamus and amygdala, This codes for the affective and recall component of pain perception, which is neither location nor intensity specific. All the centres in the brain have large projections between them, each allowing extensive modulation of the initial input. The descending pathways arise within the peri-aquaductal grey and rostro-ventral medulla, and translate inhibitory and facilitatory inputs back to the dorsal horn. The motor response generated from the cortex is not displayed.

2.4.3 **Higher brain centres**

Extensive modulation, excitation, and abnormal changes that occur in primary afferents and the dorsal horn continue throughout the higher pain centres, in particular the RVM, PAG, thalamus, primary somatosensory cortex (S1 and S2), and anterior cingulate cortex. Recent fMRI work has suggested that distinct regions of the brain are activated with noxious stimuli, pain, anticipation, recall, and emotion, and are altered in states of chronic pain. Also fMRI has allowed the study of clinical pain states and has shown extensive plasticity, remapping, and excitation, which alter pre- and post-pain control. For example, in complex regional pain syndrome (CRPS; see Chapter 8) the areas that map body location in the cortex showed a reduction in the space between them, this reverted to normal spacing when the pain had been controlled.

2.5 Interpreting pathophysiology

The more important and well-documented changes that occur following nerve damage have been reviewed and outlined. Neuropathic pain is clearly a pathological state peripherally, within the dorsal horn and higher central structures. Neuropathy is not, however, one uniform state. Some of the alterations (such as NMDA activation) probably occur in all states, others (such as sympathetic nervous system [SNS] aberrant basket formation) do not. It is appealing to think that a mechanism-based approach to the diagnosis and treatment of neuropathic pain may be here soon, however caution should be used in trying to dissect a complex, inter-dependent, plastic state into a few measurable receptors.

Key references

Carpenter, K.J. and Dickenson, A.H. (2002). Molecular aspects of pain research. *Pharmacogenomics J.*, **2**, 87–95.

Cervero, F. and Laird, J.M. (2004). Understanding the signalling and transmission of visceral nociceptive events. *J. Neurobiol.*, **61**, 45–54.

Suzuki, R. and Dickenson, A.H. (2000). Neuropathic pain: nerves bursting with excitement. *Neuroreport*, **11**, R17–21.

Suzuki, R., Rygh, L.J., and Dickenson, A.H. (2004). Bad news from the brain: descending 5-HT pathways that control spinal pain processing. *Trends Pharmacol. Sci.*, **25**, 613–17.

Tracey, I. (2005). Functional connectivity and pain: how effectively connected is your brain? *Pain*, **116**, 173–4.

Tsuda, M., Inoue, K., and Salter, M.W. (2005). Neuropathic pain and spinal microglia: a big problem from molecules in 'small' glia. *Trends Neurosci.*, **28**, 101–7.

Woolf, C.J. and Mannion, R.J. (1999). Neuropathic pain: aetiology, symptoms, mechanisms and management. *Lancet*, **353**, 1959–64.

Chapter 3

Epidemiology

Blair H. Smith and Nicola Torrance

> **Key points**
>
> - Lack of agreed definitions and diagnostic criteria for neuropathic pain hamper epidemiological studies.
> - Neuropathic pain is likely to become more common in future because of ageing populations and improved recognition.
> - Neuropathic pain probably affects around 8% of UK adults, around 24% or more of patients with long-standing diabetes, and around 20% of those who have had shingles.
> - Patients with neuropathic pain are more likely to have greater pain intensity, be older, of female gender, and of lower socio-economic status than those with other types of pain.
> - Compared with other forms of chronic pain, neuropathic pain leads to greater detrimental impact on activities of daily living and lower health-related quality of life scores.

3.1 Introduction

3.1.1 Role of epidemiology

The experience of neuropathic pain is generally more distressing than that of other forms of pain, and it can be a significant challenge for physicians to treat or control it. Epidemiology is one important discipline in the struggle to improve this situation. Epidemiology is 'the study of the distribution and determinants of health-related states … and the application of this study to the control of health problems.' It is the latter part of this definition that makes epidemiology an important clinical discipline, particularly for neuropathic pain.

3.1.2 Challenges in neuropathic pain

Keys to epidemiological study include an agreed case definition and a standardized method of case identification or ascertainment.

Unfortunately neither of these currently exists for neuropathic pain. The International Association for the Study of Pain defines it as pain 'pain arising as a direct consequence of a lesion or disease affecting the somatosensory system.' This pathophysiological definition has limited practical value for either clinical or epidemiological classification. The range of possible causes of neuropathic pain is wide and diverse, and arguments exist against classification as a single global entity.

However, others argue, and evidence suggests, that there are enough similarities between all causes of neuropathic pain in the mechanisms generating the pain, the symptoms experienced, the signs elicited and the impact on quality of life to merit detailed universal study. Most importantly, perhaps, there are similarities in the response to treatment, distinct from other types of pain. Pharmacologically, there is good evidence for different types of neuropathic pain to be considered together irrespective of aetiology.

A uniform approach to describing the epidemiology of neuropathic pain will therefore provide an understanding of the scale of the problem throughout the community (and not simply those attending the pain clinic), evidence for the development of strategies for treatment or prevention, and will allow the targeting of medical and educational resources. Good epidemiological research can also provide the basis for the design of clinical trials, including adequate power calculations.

3.2 Epidemiology of neuropathic pain as a single entity

3.2.1 Historical estimates

In 1991, a British paper suggested that the prevalence of neuropathic pain in the UK general population was probably about 1%, though this was based on estimates rather than direct evidence. A similar, though more detailed approach in the USA derived a broadly similar estimate in 1997. However, these global calculations are likely to be inaccurate, based as they are on a series of estimates of variable validity. They cannot take into consideration pain with neuropathic characteristics that has not been formally classified with one of the traditionally recognized clinical diagnoses or causes, leading to possible under-estimates. On the other hand, they may count individuals who have more than one relevant diagnosis twice, leading to possible over-estimates.

3.2.2 The need for case definition instruments

There are no agreed, standardized guidelines that allow clinicians to classify pain type (neuropathic or nociceptive) without controversy. Equally, there are no case definition instruments that can do the same for epidemiological research. This is partly because the development of these would have to be based on agreed clinical standards, but also partly because of the current debate, which suggests that many (or even most) pain diagnoses comprise a mixture of neuropathic and nociceptive mechanisms (see Chapter 1). Neuropathic pain is not necessarily a binary phenomenon i.e., present or absent, but may be a spectrum; neuropathic mechanisms may contribute a greater or lesser component to the overall aetiology of an individual's pain.

Epidemiological study is therefore most profitably aimed at identifying pain in which neuropathic features predominate, as this is where specific therapy should be targeted. Instruments have been developed based on this principle, including pain DETECT, the DN4, and the self-complete version of the Leeds Assessment of Neuropathic Symptoms and Signs (S-LANSS, see Chapter 5). These three screening instruments were developed and validated in specialist pain clinics, and have recently been used in general population studies to provide estimates of the population prevalence of pain with neuropathic features.

3.2.3 Current estimates

A recent French study used the DN4 in a postal survey of almost 24,000 adults randomly selected from a general population database. Of the responders, the study found that the population prevalence of 'chronic pain with neuropathic characteristics' was 6.9% in adults. A similar, though smaller, study in the UK used the S-LANSS and derived a similar estimate for the population prevalence of 'pain of predominantly neuropathic origin' (8.2%). This represented 17% of those with chronic pain, included a range of pain diagnoses, and was commoner among women, older respondents, and those with poorer indices of socio-economic status. The reporting of neuropathic pain was also associated with greater pain severity and health seeking behaviours. Further work is required to determine the accuracy of case identification by such screening instruments in the general population (as distinct from a pain clinic population). However, it seems that neuropathic pain in the community is more common than previously estimated.

The prevalence of neuropathic pain can be expected to increase in the future as the population ages. As well as the association with age found in the above studies, a number of causes of neuropathic pain are found to be more common in the elderly, including herpes zoster and diabetic neuropathy. Patients with chronic diseases that are associated with neuropathic pain, for example, cancer, HIV, and diabetes, are also surviving longer due to improved medical care.

3.3 Epidemiology of individual neuropathic pain syndromes

3.3.1 Painful diabetic neuropathy, postherpetic neuralgia, and neuropathic back and leg pain

Depending upon where the nerve lesion or dysfunction is located, neuropathic pain may be defined as peripheral or central, Table 3.1. It was this type of classification that led to the USA estimate of prevalence described above. The epidemiology of many of these individual diagnoses has been researched to greater or lesser extent, including the three commonest and best-understood: painful diabetic neuropathy (PDN), postherpetic neuralgia (PHN), and neuropathic back and leg pain.

Peripheral neuropathy affects perhaps a third of individuals with diabetes mellitus, though this is not always associated with pain. Depending upon the definition and severity of pain, and the type of diabetes, neuropathic pain has been found to affect between 11% and 24% of people with diabetes. The precise mechanism of pain remains unclear; so do the associations with duration and severity of diabetes, or its control, though these are all probably important. PDN is commoner in older age groups.

The lifetime prevalence of herpes zoster infection has been estimated to be 10% to 20% in the general population and as high as 50% of a cohort living to age 85 years. Of these people, between 15% and 22% have been found to develop chronic pain at the site of the shingles rash: postherpetic neuralgia. Like PDN, PHN is commoner in older people. Other risk factors include female gender, severity of shingles and associated acute pain, and psychosocial factors including distress, and living alone.

Table 3.1 Some common causes of neuropathic pain

Peripheral nerve lesion or dysfunction
- Painful diabetic neuropathy
- Post-herpetic neuralgia
- Low back pain with nerve root involvement
- Post-surgical pain (including post-mastectomy and phantom limb pain)
- Complex regional pain syndrome
- Trigeminal neuralgia
- Chemotherapy-induced neuropathy
- Neuropathy secondary to tumour infiltration

Central nerve lesion or dysfunction
- Central post-stroke pain
- Multiple sclerosis pain
- Spinal cord injury pain

Chronic low back pain is one of the commonest causes of chronic pain, with a population prevalence of up to 16%. It is frequently associated with pain caused by lumbar nerve root irritation. The painDETECT screening instrument was used in a German study of nearly 8,000 primary care attenders, and found that the 37% of individuals with low back pain were experiencing a 'predominantly neuropathic component'.

3.3.2 **Other neuropathic pain conditions**

Examples of other chronic pain conditions with neuropathic mechanisms for which we have detailed epidemiological information include:

- Post-surgical pain
- Phantom limb pain
- Central post-stroke pain
- Temperomandibular disorder pain
- Trigeminal neuralgia
- Cancer pain.

Note that these conditions are not exclusively neuropathic pain conditions. Some include a range of pain mechanisms, and others are caused by mixed nociceptive and neuropathic mechanisms. Most individuals with these conditions will have pain somewhere on the spectrum described above. A wide range of prevalence figures and risk factors is available for each of these conditions, depending on the precise definition of the condition and of pain in the studies conducted. Readers are referred to a review published by the International Association for the Study of Pain (IASP) or the detailed scientific literature available for more information.

3.3.3 **Risk factors and natural history**

Information on the long-term natural history of neuropathic pain is scant. However, from the evidence that does exist, it seems that the outlook is generally poor, with no or little change in symptoms found in follow-up studies. Once chronic neuropathic pain is established therefore, it seems to be permanent in most cases. This is consistent with our current understanding of the mechanisms of neuropathic pain, which include changes in the nervous system that are probably irreversible. Epidemiological study should therefore consider risk factors for its development, with a view to its prevention or limitation.

Common risk factors for neuropathic pain conditions found throughout the literature include older age, female gender and indices of deprivation or relatively low socio-economic status (Table 3.2). These are not modifiable, at least not by a physician, and are therefore mostly of academic or political interest, though it is worth noting the parallels with other chronic pain and non-pain conditions. A vaccine against herpes zoster is available, aiming to minimize the risk of PHN, but is not in routine use.

Table 3.2 Summary of epidemiological findings in neuropathic pain

- Affects
  - probably 6% to 8% of adults
  - around 25% or more of patients with longstanding diabetes
  - around 20% of those that have had shingles
  - around 37% of those with low back pain
- Is associated with
  - greater pain intensity than other types of pain
  - older age
  - female gender
  - lower socioeconomic status
- Compared with other forms of chronic pain, leads to
  - greater impact on daily living
  - lower quality of life scores

Of greater clinical interest, perhaps, are the psychosocial risk factors (such as the association between distress and PHN), as well as some clinical factors specific for each condition. These may be amenable to intervention, and therefore prevention or limitation of neuropathic pain.

Research is still required in this area, but several findings show promise. For example, less intense post-mastectomy pain in the acute phase after surgery may be associated with reduced chronic neuropathic pain. Prevention should therefore focus on the immediate post-operative phase, though this requires detailed confirmation. Counselling or other psychological interventions aimed at the reduction of distress might also be effective in reducing chronic pain after surgery or amputation. Again, confirmation is required through clinical trials, and these are active or planned in several locations.

3.4 Impact of neuropathic pain

3.4.1 Quality of life measures

Although there is a lack of general population research in this area, studies consistently find that individuals with neuropathic pain conditions have poorer health than those without, in every health dimension measured: physical, psychological, and social. They also have more severe, unpleasant pain than those with other types of chronic pain. This research confirms clinical impressions, and tells us that these patients have greater disruption of daily activity, poorer sleep and quality of life, and poorer mental health than they would if their pain could be adequately treated. This could be said of any chronic pain, but seems to be particularly true for neuropathic pain.

The Neuropathic Pain Scale (NPS, see Chapter 5) was developed to measure specific characteristics of the experience of chronic pain. It includes sub-scales measuring the pain's intensity, heat, sharpness, hypersensitivity, and unpleasantness, all of which score higher among people with neuropathic pain than with other pain types. The fact that these sub-scales are sensitive to change, and their scores improve with treatment (such as gabapentin or lidocaine patches) confirms the benefits of intervention. Several studies have also shown improvements in measures of general physical, psychological and social well-being as secondary outcomes of interventions for neuropathic pain. Further research is required in the general population to establish baseline and natural history data.

3.5 **Further epidemiological research**

3.5.1 **Need for consensus on definitions**

Further advances in the epidemiological understanding of neuropathic pain are hampered by the absence of agreed detailed definitions and diagnostic criteria for classifying neuropathic pain. If and when these are established, standard instruments can be developed for case identification and ascertainment in research. Until then, our information must continue to be drawn from studies of specific conditions with neuropathic mechanisms of pain (such as PDN), or from pragmatic approximations (such as 'pain of predominantly neuropathic origin'). To a certain extent the current debate about the mechanisms and binary nature of neuropathic pain will need to be resolved before these gold standards can be designed and accepted widely. However, this must not hamper clinical progress unduly.

3.5.2 **Improving prevention and management strategies**

The important outcome of epidemiological research in neuropathic pain, as with all other conditions, is the further development of prevention and management strategies. If these are successful, a great deal of suffering will be relieved.

Existing epidemiological tools such as the S-LANSS and DN4 have an important place, but need further validation, particularly in general population settings. This will allow large-scale population-based research, and a clearer understanding of the aetiology, incidence, risk factors and natural history associated with chronic neuropathic pain.

This information is crucial in the design of prevention strategies, or of interventions designed to minimize disability and maximize capacity. It is also important in the design of the clinical trials to which the epidemiological research must all lead, including targeting interventions, identifying important outcome measures, and powering studies with appropriate sample sizes. A particularly exciting possibility is the study of biological mechanisms (including genetic factors) in the development of neuropathic pain, and there are several large population studies underway internationally that may eventually allow this.

Key references

Bouhassira D., Lanteri-Minet M., Attal N., Laurent B., Touboul C. (2008). Prevalence of chronic pain with neuropathic characteristics in the general population. *Pain*, **136**, 380–7.

Bowsher D. (1991). Neurogenic pain syndromes and their management. *Br Med Bull*, **47**, 644–66.

Crombie I.K., Croft P.R., Linton S.J., LeResche L., Von Korff M. (eds) (1999). *Epidemiology of Pain*. IASP Press, Seattle.

Dworkin R.H. (2002). An overview of neuropathic pain: syndromes, symptoms, signs, and several mechanisms. *Clin J Pain*, **18**, 343–9.

Freynhagen R., Baron R., Gockel U., Tolle T.R. (2006). painDETECT a new screening questionnaire to identify neuropathic components in patients with back pain. *Curr Med Res Opin*, **22**, 1911–20.

Hansson P.T., Dickenson A.H. (2005). Pharmacological treatment of peripheral neuropathic pain conditions on shared commonalities despite multiple etiologies. *Pain*, **113**, 251–4.

Jensen M.P., Chodroff M.J., Dworkin R.H. (2007). The impact of neuropathic pain on health-related quality of life: review and implications. *Neurol.*, **68**, 1178–82.

Sadosky A., McDermott A.M., Brandenburg N.A., Strauss M. (2008). A review of the epidemiology of painful diabetic peripheral neuropathy, postherpetic neuralgia, and less commonly studied neuropathic pain conditions. *Pain Practice*, **8**, 45–56.

Schmader K.E. (2002). Epidemiology and impact on quality of life of postherpetic neuralgia and painful diabetic neuropathy. *Clin J Pain*, **18**, 350–4.

Torrance N., Smith B.H., Bennett M.I., Lee A.J. (2006). The epidemiology of chronic pain of predominantly neuropathic origin. Results from a general population study. *J Pain*, **7**, 281–9.

Chapter 4

Clinical assessment and diagnostic work-up

Roman Rolke

Key points

- Neuropathic pain arises as a direct consequence of a lesion or disease affecting the somatosensory system
- The diagnostic work-up of neuropathic pain syndromes includes information on the patient's history and a bedside examination focussed on the main questions:
- Is the distribution of pain and sensory deficit neuroanatomically logical?
- Is the disease history suggestive of a relevant lesion or disease to the peripheral or central somatosensory system?
- Common neuropathic pain symptoms are spontaneous pain (ongoing pain without detectable stimulation) and evoked pains (abnormal responses to stimulation)
- Clinical signs such as hyperalgesia, allodynia, or hypoalgesia and hypoesthesia may indicate possible underlying neurobiological pain mechanisms such as peripheral/central sensitization or deafferentation of the nociceptive system
- Conventional electrophysiology (nerve conduction studies and somatosensory-evoked potentials) are objective measures mainly confirming a large fibre sensory deficit. Small fibre function usually escapes these conventional methods
- Quantitative sensory testing (QST) is the analysis of the subjective response to a somatosensory perception after external stimuli of controlled intensity. Using QST it is possible to assess both small fibre function as well as positive and negative sensory phenomena.

4.1 **Re-defining neuropathic pain**

Neuropathic pain arises as a direct consequence of a lesion or disease affecting the somatosensory system. Neuropathic pain is distinct from nociceptive pain in the way that the latter is induced by activation of nociceptive nerve endings without neural damage. In clinical practice it is important to assess location, quality, and intensity of pain. Neuropathy is plausible, whenever sensory abnormalities both painless and painful fit to a neuroanatomically logical distribution. However, neural damage does not necessarily indicate the presence of neuropathic pain, since patients with neuropathy may also suffer from psychogenic or other nociceptive pains such as headache, musculoskeletal, arthritic, or cancer pain. The degree of certainty regarding the presence of neuropathic pain reflects the overlapping evidence from clinical bedside examination, pain drawings, pain questionnaires, laboratory tests such as conventional electrophysiology, and quantitative sensory testing. This thorough diagnostic work-up allows the performance of all relevant somatosensory submodalities to be tested, including both peripheral nerve fibres and spinal pathways to the corresponding brain centres.

4.2 **Symptoms in neuropathic pain patients**

The most prominent symptom in neuropathic pain is spontaneous pain. Spontaneous pain may be continuous with varying or stable intensity, or intermittent with paroxysmal, frequently electric shock like attacks. This type of pain may be induced by pathological spontaneous activity of damaged neurons in the absence of a detectable stimulus. However, in some neuropathic pain conditions such as trigeminal neuralgia, ongoing pain is missing. Instead evoked pain may occur after speaking, chewing or touching the face.

Non-painful paraesthesias may be also present in neuropathic patients alongside painful sensations. For example, patients with diabetic neuropathy frequently report pricking or tingling sensations in the feet that do not hurt. These paraesthesias most likely reflect spontaneous activity of large myelinated $A\beta$ fibres that normally mediate the sensation of touch or vibration.

4.3 **Clinical signs and possible underlying neurobiological mechanisms**

Increasing evidence from animal research and human (surrogate) pain models suggested a link between clinical signs and neurobiological mechanisms. However, the mechanisms underlying some of the clinical signs in neuropathic pain are under debate and so the idea of a mechanism-based classification of neuropathic pain in clinical practice is an ongoing research controversy. Table 4.1 illustrates some clinical signs in relation to possible underlying pathophysiology. In summary, positive and negative sensory signs exist. Positive sensory signs indicate a sensitization of peripheral or central nociceptive channels, while negative signs point to a loss of sensory function that may be due to neural damage or reduced/inhibited central processing of the peripheral input.

As Table 4.1 shows, different neurobiological mechanisms exist that may be present in isolation or in combination in one and the same pain patient. Peripheral and central sensitizations of nociceptive channels are universal mechanisms shared by all types of nociceptive pains and neuropathic pain as well. However, the mechanism of deafferentation (damage to the nerve causing loss of afferent input) is only present in neuropathic pain, when neural lesion or disease have occurred.

4.4 Neuropathic pain—definite, probable or possible

Previously, neuropathic pain was considered as binary phenomena: either present or absent. Recently, a grade of certainty for the diagnosis of neuropathic pain has been proposed and this depends on the patient's disease history, clinical examination, and supporting evidence from other confirming laboratory or objective testing procedures.

4.4.1 Criteria to be evaluated for the diagnosis of neuropathic pain:

1. Pain with a distinct neuroanatomically plausible distribution?
2. A history suggestive of a relevant lesion or disease affecting the peripheral or central somatosensory system?
3. Demonstration of the distinct neuroanatomically plausible distribution by at least one confirmatory test?
4. Demonstration of the relevant lesion or disease by at least one confirmatory test?

4.4.2 Grading of certainty for the presence of neuropathic pain:

- Definite neuropathic pain: all criteria fulfilled (1 to 4);
- Probable neuropathic pain: 1 and 2, plus either 3 or 4;
- Possible neuropathic pain: 1 and 2, without confirmatory evidence from 3 or 4.

Table 4.1 Clinical signs, bedside examination, and possible underlying neurobiological mechanisms

Selection of signs	Definition	Bedside examination to test for the presence of positive or negative signs	Possible involved neurobiological mechanism		
			Deafferentation	Peripheral sensitization	Central sensitization
			Sensitivity to stimuli during bedside examination		
Positive signs					
Hyperalgesia	Increased pain sensitivity[a]				
to heat	... of the skin	Painful hot thermo roller/ test-tube	↓	↑↑	↓?
to cold	... of the skin	Painful cold thermo roller/ test-tube	↓	↑	↑?
to pinprick	... of the skin	Toothpick, pin	↓	↑?	↑↑
to blunt pressure	... of deeper tissues	Examiner's thumb	↓	↑?	↓↑?
Allodynia[b]	Pain in response to a non-nociceptive stimulus[a]	Brush, cotton swab, cotton wisp/wool tip	↑	↑	↓

Negative signs

Hypoesthesia (thermal/mechanical/other)	Reduced sensitivity to non-painful stimuli	Cold reflex hammer, cold and warm thermo rollers/test-tubes Q-tip, tuning fork, brush, cotton swab, examiner's hand	→	↑	↑, ↑[c]
Hypoalgesia (thermal/mechanical/other)	Reduced sensitivity to painful stimuli	Painful cold and hot thermo rollers/test-tubes, toothpick, pin, thumb of investigator	→	↑	↑

This Table is modified from Woolf and Mannion 1999, Hansson et al. 2007.

↑, increased sensitivity to bedside examination stimulus, ↓, decreased sensitivity, →, sensitivity not altered or not exploitable, ?, not sufficiently tested or described in some studies, still under debate.

[a] New IASP definitions (Loeser and Treede 2008), IASP = International Association for the Study of Pain.

[b] This term should only be used, when it is known that the test stimulus does not activate nociceptors. Dynamic tactile allodynia to stroking light touch, e.g. brushing the skin, is the only established example (IASP 2008).

[c] Secondary tactile hypoesthesia has been described within the presence of central sensitization (Magerl and Treede 2004).

4.5 **Bedside examination**

Bedside examination should include location, quality, and intensity of pain. During this examination information on both spontaneous and evoked pains as well as all relevant clinical symptoms and signs should be recorded. A detailed neurological examination is invaluable in the detection of neuropathic signs in response to neural damage and should include assessment of sensory and motor function, reflexes, and autonomic functions such as skin perfusion or sweating. The most important aspect of this bedside investigation is the sensory examination. Sensory deficits should be neuroanatomically consistent before concluding the presence of neuropathic pain and so pain drawings may be helpful to map the pain distribution. Using simple equipment it is possible to assess both different types of sensory nerve fibres and their respective central (spinal cord/brainstem) channels to the brain. For example, using a cold reflex hammer it is possible to compare the sensation of cold between the painful and a mirror image control area. This type of non-painful stimulus is mediated by thinly myelinated Aδ fibres that project to the brain via the anterolateral aspects of the spinal cord (spinothalamic tract). Accordingly, a reduced sensation of cold may occur due to a lesion along this neuroanatomical axis up to the brain. The same applies for the sensation of warmth that is mediated by unmyelinated C fibres. Warmth sensitivity can be assessed using warm thermo rollers or test-tubes. Heat and cold pain as well as all other mechanically evoked pains are also mediated by other C or Aδ fibres that project to the brain via the spinothalamic tract of the spinal cord.

In contrast, the non-painful mechanical sensation of touch or vibration is mediated by thickly myelinated Aβ fibres that project to the brain via the lemniscal system that is located in the dorsal aspects of the spinal cord. For example, using a cotton wool tip to test for the sensation of static light touch, or pins to test for the sensation of pricking sharp pain, it is easily possible to assess both peripheral Aβ and Aδ fibres functions as well as the performance of the lemniscal or spinothalamic projections of the spinal cord to the brain. While bedside examination allows a qualitative estimate of sensory functions, this performance can be quantified using quantitative sensory testing (QST). Table 4.2 shows details on peripheral nerve fibres, central pathways and bedside as well QST devices that may be involved when examining the sensation of different thermal or mechanical stimuli.

Table 4.2 Assessment of somatosensory modalities including peripheral and central pathways as well as test devices

Type of stimulus	Peripheral sensory channel	Spinal/brainstem pathway	Bedside examination	QST
Thermal				
Cold	Aδ fibres	Spinothalamic	Cold reflex hammer,	Computer controlled
Warmth	C fibres	Spinothalamic	Cold and warm or hot	thermal testing device
Heat pain	C, Aδ fibres	Spinothalamic	thermo rollers/ test-tubes	
Cold pain	C, Aδ fibres	Spinothalamic		
Mechanical				
Blunt pressure	Aδ, C fibres	Spinothalamic	Examiner's thumb	Algometer
Pinprick	Aδ, C fibres	Spinothalamic	Toothpick, pin	Calibrated pins/ pinpricks
Static light touch	Aβ fibres	Lemniscal	Cotton wool tip	Calibrated von Frey hairs
Brushing	Aβ fibres	Lemniscal	Brush, cotton swab	Brush, cotton wisp/ wool tip
Vibration	Aβ fibres	Lemniscal	Tuning fork	Calibrated tuning fork, vibrameter

Modified from Hansson et al. 2007.
QST, quantitative sensory testing.

4.6 Quantitative sensory testing (QST)

QST is the standardized and formalized extension of the clinical neurological examination of sensory function using controlled (calibrated) stimuli. QST is a subjective (psychophysical) method that requires cooperation of the patient being investigated. QST mimics the natural environment using thermal, mechanical or chemical stimuli that test for the performance of the somatosensory system from the peripheral receptors located at nerve fibre terminals in the skin up to the brain. Additionally, electrical stimuli have been used that exert excitation of nociceptive (C, Aδ fibres) as well as non-nociceptive nerve fibres (Aβ) bypassing the different thermal, mechanical, or chemical receptors on the fibre terminals. Using the latter approach, sensitization of such receptors is not exploitable using electrical stimulation.

To measure the sensitivity of a patient to stimuli of a given intensity, thresholds can be quantified. The 'method of *levels*' is a time consuming approach that repetitively offers stimuli below and above the assumed thresholds. The final detection threshold represents the intensity, where 50% of stimuli can be detected. For example, the tactile detection threshold to von Frey-filaments (Figure 4.1) represents the applied force that was detected in 50% of repetitive skin contacts with this non-painful stimulus. The same applies for the pain threshold that is usually defined as the stimulus intensity that begins to be painful in 50% of repetitive stimuli. The pain tolerance threshold is the highest intensity of a painful stimulus that a subject is willing to tolerate. Another psychophysical method is the 'method of *limits*', where the detection and pain thresholds are defined as the first detected or painful stimulus within rising stimulus intensity, e.g., within increasing temperature of a computer controlled thermotester. This method is much faster. However, in contrast to the 'method of levels' thresholds are overestimated, since the final threshold always includes a reaction time artefact.

Figure 4.1 Von Frey-filament touching the skin

As with bedside testing, QST provides a large set of sensory examination procedures that allow testing of all relevant submodalities of the somatosensory system (peripheral receptors, C, Aδ, Aβ fibres, central pathways to the brain; Table 4.2). Moreover, increase or decrease of thresholds reflects possible underlying neurobiological mechanisms (Table 1). For example, the mechanical pain threshold to pinprick stimuli has found to be reduced (i.e., the sensitivity to pinprick is increased) in animal and human (surrogate) models of central nociceptive sensitization (Figure 4.2). More accepted is the presence of dynamic mechanical allodynia (DMA) to stroking light touch with a brush or cotton wisp to reflect this central nociception sensitization as well.

Present recommendations, however, do not advise taking QST abnormalities as conclusive demonstration of a neuropathic pain. QST as well as other laboratory tests are time consuming and some of the equipment is very expensive. Thus, so far QST plays a major role in clinical research studies that focus on both the investigation of small fibre function that escapes conventional electrophysiology, as well as the detection of positive sensory phenomena resulting from peripheral or central nociceptive sensitizations.

4.7 Objective laboratory testing procedures

Sensory nerve conduction studies and somatosensory-evoked potentials (SEP) represent the most essential part of conventional electrophysiology to support the diagnosis of neuropathic pain in the clinical practice. However, both electrical stimulation methods bypass the receptors adjacent to the nerve fibre terminals in the skin and test mainly for the performance of thickly myelinated Aβ fibres. Laser-evoked potentials (LEP) close this gap by stimulating Aδ as well as C fibres of the skin resulting in brain activity that can be recorded similar to a SEP. Microneurography is only available in a few specialized centres and this technique allows the function of all relevant sensory nerve fibres, including the peripheral performance of C and Aδ fibres, to be characterised. In contrast to microneurography, sensory nerve conduction studies, SEPs and LEPs are non-invasive. Another invasive procedure is the sampling of skin biopsies that gives detailed information on the numbers of small epidermal nerve fibres that may be reduced in neuropathic pain.

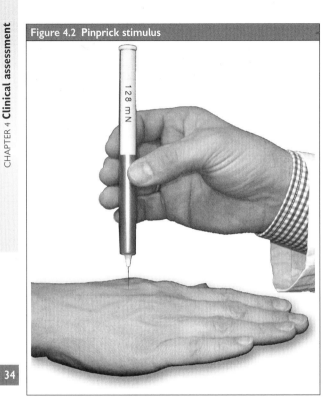

Figure 4.2 Pinprick stimulus

Key references

Cruccu, G., Anand, P., Attal, N., Garcia-Larrea, L., Haanpää, M., Jørum, E., et al. (2004). EFNS guidelines on neuropathic pain assessment. *Eur. J. Neurol.*, **11**, 153–62.

Hansson, P., Backonja, M., Bouhassira, D. (2007). Usefulness and limitations of quantitative sensory testing: clinical and research application in neuropathic pain states. *Pain*, **129**, 256–9.

Loeser, J.D., Treede, R.-D. (2008). The Kyoto protocol of IASP Basic Pain Terminology. *Pain*, **137**, 473–7.

Magerl, W., Treede, R.-D. (2004). Secondary tactile hypoesthesia: a novel type of pain-induced somatosensory plasticity in human subjects. *Neurosci. Lett.*, **361**, 136–9.

Rolke, R., Baron, R., Maier, C., Tölle, T.R., Treede, R.-D., Beyer, A., Binder, A., *et al.* (2006). Quantitative sensory testing in the German Research Network on Neuropathic Pain (DFNS): standardized protocol and reference values. *Pain*, **123**, 231–43.

Treede, R.-D., Jensen, T.S., Campbell, J.N., Cruccu, G., Dostrovsky, J.O., Griffin, J.W., Hansson P, *et al.* (2008). Neuropathic pain: redefinition and a grading system for clinical and research purposes. *Neurology, **70**, 1630–5.

Woolf, C.J., Mannion, R.J. (1999). Neuropathic pain: aetiology, symptoms, mechanisms, and management. *Lancet*, **353**, 1959–64.

Chapter 5

Screening tools and measurement tools for neuropathic pain

Michael I. Bennett

> ### Key points
>
> - Verbal description differs between neuropathic and nociceptive pain and can contribute important information to the assessment process
> - Screening tools alert the clinician to the possible presence of neuropathic pain mechanisms but they do not replace clinical diagnosis
> - Measurement tools assess the intensity of particular qualities of neuropathic pain once a diagnosis has been made
> - Screening tools are probably most useful in identifying potential neuropathic pain in non-specialist settings, particularly primary care
> - Both types of tools can improve measurement sensitivity within clinical trials and epidemiological research which allows more direct comparisons between studies and helps to identify pain qualities that might respond to specific therapies.

5.1 Role of verbal description

Classical or textbook lists of symptoms and signs make for an easy diagnosis. The problem in practice is that most patients are not textbooks and the presentation of most disease, and pain in particular, takes some analysis.

As pain remains a subjective phenomenon and neuropathic pain is thought to result in unique sensations, it makes sense to use verbal description as a basis for distinguishing neuropathic pain from tissue injury pain. A number of studies have shown that patients with neuropathic pain select certain pain descriptors with more frequency than those with nociceptive pain. This led to the development of several scales to systematically assess this information.

These scales can be divided into screening tools and measurement tools. Screening tools alert the clinician to the possible presence of neuropathic pain mechanisms; they are not diagnostic tools. Measurement tools assess the intensity of particular qualities of neuropathic pain once a diagnosis has been made. Both types of tools rely on verbal description (sometimes with simple bedside examination) and they can contribute important information to the assessment process alongside clinical history, examination, and investigation (see Chapter 4).

Alongside qualitative verbal description, generic information on pain intensity (such as visual analogue scores) and its impact on daily living (often called 'interference') also form part of the patient assessment in neuropathic pain. These aspects are not discussed in detail here.

5.2 Screening tools

5.2.1 Leeds Assessment of Neuropathic Symptoms and Signs (LANSS) pain scale

The LANSS was the first published screening tool that attempted to discriminate between neuropathic pain and nociceptive pain. In this regard, it has around 80% accuracy when compared to expert clinician assessment. The LANSS consists of five symptom items and two clinical examination items (allodynia and pinprick testing), and takes around five minutes to complete. The LANSS has been used extensively in the UK and internationally and has been validated in a number of independent studies examining cancer neuropathic pain, fibromyalgia, low back pain, and pain clinic populations.

Although the LANSS was not designed as a measurement tool, it has also shown sensitivity to treatment effects: for example, patients with intractable neuropathic pain (trigeminal neuralgia or post-stroke pain) showed reduction in LANSS score after successful treatment with transcranial magnetic stimulation, but not with placebo.

The LANSS has been further developed into a patient self-report tool, the S-LANSS score (see Appendix 2). Positive scores on the LANSS or S-LANSS identify patients with pain of predominantly neuropathic origin (POPNO) i.e., pain that is dominated by neuropathic mechanisms.

5.2.2 Douleur Neuropathique en 4 questions (DN4)

The DN4 was developed and validated in French using 160 patients with either neuropathic or nociceptive pain. It consists of 7 items related to symptoms and 3 related to clinical examination; a total score of 4 or more out of 10 suggests neuropathic pain. Compared with clinical diagnosis, the DN4 showed 83% sensitivity and 90% specificity in the development study. The DN4 can be used as self-report questionnaire using the 7 symptom items only.

5.2.3 painDETECT

This screening tool was developed and validated in German and is a patient-based (self-report) questionnaire with 9 items that do not require a clinical examination. There are 7 weighted sensory descriptor items (rated never to very strongly) and 2 items that describe the spatial (radiating) and temporal characteristics of the individual pain pattern. painDETECT was originally developed to distinguish neuropathic low back pain from non-neuropathic low back pain (see Chapter 10). The tool correctly classified 83% of patients with a sensitivity of 85% and a specificity of 80%.

5.2.4 Neuropathic Pain Questionnaire (NPQ)

The NPQ consists of 12 items that include 10 related to sensations or sensory responses, and 2 related to affect. It was developed in a large population of patients with a broad range of chronic pain diagnoses. The NPQ demonstrated 66% sensitivity and 74% specificity compared to clinical diagnosis in the validation sample. The short form of the NPQ maintained similar discriminative properties with only 3 items (numbness, tingling and pain increase in response to touch).

5.2.5 ID-Pain

ID-Pain was developed in the USA and consists of five sensory descriptor items and one item relating to whether pain is located in the joints (used to identify nociceptive pain). It is a tool that does not require a clinical examination. The tool was developed in a chronic pain population that included nociceptive, mixed or neuropathic etiology. A cut-off score of 3 or more on ID-Pain suggests the possible presence of a neuropathic component to the patient's pain. In validation studies, 22% of the nociceptive group, 39% of the mixed group, and 58% of the neuropathic group scored above this cut off.

5.2.6 Screening tool content

All five of these screening tools make use of similar language to discriminate patients with neuropathic pain from those with other types of chronic pain with up to 80% sensitivity and specificity (see Table 5.1). This is powerful evidence for the reliability and validity of this approach even though these tools were developed by different researchers in different countries with varying approaches to validation and testing. Further validation of these standardized tools is needed across cultures and languages by other researchers to reach consensus on which tool is most suited for a particular context or task.

Table 5.1 Comparison of screening tools content

Symptoms	LANSS[a]	DN4[a]	NPQ	pain-DETECT	ID Pain
Pricking, tingling, pins and needles	●	●	●	●	●
Electric shocks or shooting	●	●	●	●	●
Hot or burning	●	●	●	●	●
Numbness		●	●	●	●
Pain evoked by light touching	●		●	●	●
Painful cold or freezing pain		●	●		
Pain evoked by mild pressure				●	
Pain evoked by heat or cold				●	
Pain evoked by changes in weather			●		
Pain limited to joints[b]					○
Itching		●			
Temporal patterns				●	
Radiation of pain				●	
Autonomic changes	●				
Clinical Examination					
Brush allodynia	●	●			
Raised soft touch threshold		●			
Raised pin prick threshold	●	●			

a = tools that involve clinical examination
b = used to identify non-neuropathic pain

5.3 **Measurement tools**

5.3.1 **Neuropathic pain scale (NPS)**

This was the first scale to measure the intensity of 11 features that were thought to be reflective of neuropathic pain. These included generic features such as overall pain intensity, unpleasantness, and periodicity (intermittent, constant, flare-ups) as well as more specific features such as sharp, itchy, burning, and surface pain. The scale was not intended to distinguish neuropathic pain from nociceptive pain but has been widely used to measure changes in intensity of neuropathic pain symptoms. In particular, the NPS has shown sensitivity to treatment effects.

5.3.2 **Neuropathic Pain Symptom Inventory**

This measurement tool was developed by the same French group that later produced the DN4. It includes 10 descriptors (plus two temporal items) that allow discrimination and quantification of five distinct clinically relevant dimensions of neuropathic pain syndromes. The psychometric properties of the NPSI suggest that it might be used to characterize subgroups of neuropathic pain patients and verify whether they respond differentially to various pharmacological agents or other therapeutic interventions.

5.4 **Applications in clinical practice and research**

5.4.1 **Screening tools do not replace clinical assessment**

The purpose of screening tools is to identify patients with neuropathic pain based on a few key symptoms and signs. This design necessarily emphasizes commonalities of neuropathic pain conditions while neglecting their diversity. One potential consequence of this approach is that it may miss patients with unusual presentations of neuropathic pain. The evidence from the validation studies detailed above shows that in general, these tools fail to identify about 10–20% of patients with clinician diagnosed neuropathic pain (and misdiagnose a similar proportion with nociceptive pain).

This might be an issue of screening tool failure, lack of unique verbal description by these patients or inconsistent diagnostic practice, or all of these. It is therefore important to note that although screening tools offer guidance for further diagnostic evaluation (including clinical examination) and pain management, they do not replace clinical judgment in the assessment of an individual patient's pain.

5.4.2 **Identifying potential neuropathic pain in non-specialist settings**

The debate that surrounds the definition of neuropathic pain (see Chapters 1 and 4) will continue for some time to come. Until consensus is agreed on a diagnostic approach to neuropathic pain, screening tools can help to identify potential patients with neuropathic pain and this is probably their chief clinical strength. They are likely to be particularly helpful in non-specialist settings such as primary care.

Their ease of use by non-specialists and by patients themselves, in clinic or via telephone or computer, makes these screening tools ideal for providing immediate descriptive information. This can then alert clinicians to undertake further assessment, which may subsequently influence management decisions.

5.4.3 **Improving sensitivity in clinical measurement**

Traditionally, research studies on neuropathic pain have used clinician assessment as the gold standard reference but significant variance between, and within, clinicians makes study populations difficult to compare. In addition, lack of detail about specific symptoms, and patterns of symptoms, obscures potentially useful information.

Screening tools and measurement tools can help standardize assessment approaches to patients with neuropathic pain in clinical and research contexts. This in turn might allow better identification of which components of a patient's pain respond better to specific therapeutic strategies.

These tools can also be used as standardized case identification tools in epidemiological studies, and this is probably their chief research strength. Good data from these types of studies has been lacking but studies have recently been reported using the S-LANSS and DN4 (see Chapter 3) and this is helping to progress understanding of the clinical impact of neuropathic pain and associated features.

Key references

Bennett, M. (2001). The LANSS pain scale: the Leeds Assessment of Neuropathic Symptoms and Signs. *Pain*, **92**, 147–57.

Bennett M.I., Attal N., Backonja M.M., Baron R., Bouhassira D., Freynhagen R., Scholz J., Tolle T., Wittchen H., Jensen T.S. (2007). Using screening tools to identify neuropathic pain (Topical Review). *Pain*, **127**, 199–203.

Bennett M.I., Bouhassira D. (2007). Epidemiology of neuropathic pain: can we use the screening tools? (editorial) *Pain*, **132**, 12–13.

Bennett, M.I., Smith, B.H., Torrance, N., Potter, J. (2005). The S-LANSS score for identifying pain of predominantly neuropathic origin: validation for use in clinic and postal research. *J. Pain*, **6**, 149–58.

Bouhassira D., Attal N., Fermanian J., Alchaar H., Gautron M., Masquelier E., Rostaing S., Lanteri-Minet M., Collin E., Grisart J., Boureau F. (2004). Development and validation of the Neuropathic Pain Symptom Inventory. *Pain*, **108**, 248–57.

Bouhassira D., Attal N., Alchaar H., Boureau F., Bruxelle J., Cunin G., *et al.* (2005). Comparison of pain syndromes associated with nervous or somatic lesions and development of a new neuropathic pain diagnostic questionnaire (DN4). *Pain*, **114**, 29–36.

Freynhagen R., Baron R., Gockel U., Tolle T. (2006). painDetect: a new screeing questionnaire to detect neuropathic components in patients with back pain. *Curr Med Res Opin*, **22**, 1911–20.

Galer, B.S. and Jensen, M.P. (1997). Development and preliminary validation of a pain measure specific to neuropathic pain: the Neuropathic Pain Scale. *Neurology*, **48**, 332–8.

Krause S.J., Backonja M.M. (2003). Development of a Neuropathic Pain Questionnaire. *Clin J Pain*, **19**, 306–14.

Portenoy R. for the ID Pain Steering Committee (2006). Development and testing of a neuropathic pain screening questionnaire: ID Pain. *Curr Med Res Opin*, **22**, 1555–65.

Chapter 6

Peripheral neuropathic pain

Tim Nash

Key points

- Damage to peripheral nerves, including cranial nerves and spinal nerve roots, can result in peripheral neuropathic pain
- Speed of onset and associated symptoms and signs can point towards possible causes
- Common conditions include diabetic neuropathy, post-herpetic neuralgia, and post-surgical neuropathies including phantom limb pain
- Less common conditions result from Guillain-Barré syndrome, deficiency states, and toxic neuropathies
- Treatment is based on co-analgesics with or without opioids. Some conditions, such as trigeminal neuralgia and other compression problems, can respond well to decompression surgery.

6.1 Introduction

6.1.1 Role of peripheral nociceptive system

It is a commonly held belief that the pain system has an important role in alerting the individual to the threat of tissue damage. Pain is not normally felt until after the injury has occurred, and frequently not until some time after the injury. It is therefore questionable as to whether pain has any value. Neuropathic pain particularly has no value, the pain developing and persisting as a result of damage to or dysfunction of the nervous system, persisting after all possible healing has occurred.

6.1.2 Sites of peripheral damage

Peripheral neuropathic pain can result from any damage to or dysfunction of the peripheral nervous system, which includes the cranial nerves (except the optic nerve), spinal nerve roots, dorsal root ganglia, peripheral nerve trunks, and nerve terminals. Disruption of the somatosensory system results in loss of sensation and analgesia in the affected area. This can affect motor, sensory, autonomic, or mixed nerve fibres, and may lead to aberrant somatosensory processing, with the paradox of pain in the hypo-aesthetic area (see Chapter 2).

6.1.3 Painless neuropathies

Neuropathies such as leprosy, congenital insensitivity to pain (Hereditary Sensory and Autonomic Neuropathy), and Tangier disease (familial high protein density lipoprotein deficiency), are painless because of the predominant loss of pain sensation. A common misconception is that it is this absence of pain sensation that often leads to severe mutilation. Sternbach pointed out in 1963 that where other sensory cues persisted in patients with congenital insensitivity to pain, they were able to avoid such harm.

6.2 Clinical manifestations

6.2.1 Symptoms and history

Despite the varied conditions, site, and type of nerve damage, the clinical picture in peripheral neuropathic pain is generally very similar (see also Chapter 4).

The pain may include the following features:

- It may be spontaneous, and can be paroxysmal, lasting for seconds up to minutes, several times a day to a few times every week
- Paroxysmal pain may be shooting, intense, or sharp
- It may be constantly burning, aching, or sore
- Typically there is also evoked pain, mostly caused by lightly touching the skin or by exposure to wind (allodynia)
- Frequently dysaesthesia (numbness, pins and needles) is present.

The pain may vary spontaneously, but typically intensifies with activity and exposure to cold. There may be increased sympathetic activity.

Common features of peripheral neuropathic pain include a history of:

- Possible neurological injury (surgery or trauma)
- Spontaneous or paroxysmal pain
- Pain in distribution of a nerve (neuralgia)
- Pain persisting after tissue healing
- Descriptors such as burning, electrical, shooting, stabbing
- Poor response to opioids, with steadily increasing opioid requirement.

The speed of onset of the neuropathy can give a guide as to its aetiology (Table 6.1).

Table 6.1 Likely causes of neuropathy according to speed of onset	
Acute onset	Inflammatory
	Immunological
	Toxic
	Vascular
Subacute onset over weeks or months	Toxic
	Nutritional
	Systemic disease
Chronic onset over many years	Hereditary
	Metabolic disease

6.2.2 Clinical examination of peripheral nerves

This should assess the presence of:

- Allodynia (pain elicited by a stimulus that does not normally provoke pain)
- Hyperpathia (abnormally painful reaction to a stimulus, especially a repeated stimulus, often explosive, radiating, and with after-sensations)
- Hypoaesthesia (decreased sensitivity to stimulation)
- Hyperaesthesia (increased sensitivity to stimulation)
- Hypoalgesia (diminished pain in response to a normally painful stimulus)
- Hyperalgesia (increased pain in response to a normally painful stimulus)
- Paraesthesia (unpleasant abnormal sensation, spontaneous or provoked)
- Neurological deficit (e.g. nerve root avulsion)
- Autonomic/vasomotor dysfunction (e.g. unilateral skin temperature changes)
- Tinel's sign (tapping damaged peripheral nerves, causes shocks radiating in nerve distribution).

Establishing a diagnosis may enable treatment of the cause and consequent improvement in the pain. Diagnostic tests for peripheral neuropathic pain are summarized in Table 6.2.

Examination findings may suggest that the peripheral neuropathy is symmetrical or asymmetrical and this can point towards possible causes (Tables 6.3 and 6.4).

Table 6.2 Tests used to aid diagnosis of peripheral neuropathies

Diagnostic test	Investigates	Establishes
Nerve conduction and Electromyography	Large-fibre function only	Nerve disorder: • generalized polyneuropathy • multifocal neuropathy • mononeuropathy • distinguishes between primary demyelinating neuropathy and axonal neuropathy
Quantitative sensory testing	Nerve fibre function: • small myelinated • small unmyelinated • large myelinated	Can particularly show pure small-fibre neuropathy
Blood tests	Blood sugar Vitamin assays Lead and other assays Immunoglobulins and anti-neural antibody	Metabolic disease Nutritional deficiency Toxicity states Immune-mediated neuropathies
Genetic screening		Inherited neuropathies
Cerebrospinal fluid assessment	Protein Cellular response	Radicular or meningeal involvement
Nerve and muscle biopsy	Nerve/muscle pathology	Mononeuritis multiplex: • vasculitis • amyloidosis • leprosy • subacute or chronic distal symmetric polyneuropathies Genetically determined paediatric disorders

Table 6.3 Pathological causes of symmetrical painful neuropathies and neuropathic pain	
Metabolic	Impaired glucose tolerance Diabetes mellitus Hypoglycaemic (insulinoma) Hypothyroidism
Nutritional/deficiency	Pellagra (niacin deficiency) Beriberi (thiamine deficiency) Multiple nutritional deficiencies
Toxic	Drugs: • alcohol • antiretroviral drugs • cytotoxic • isoniazid, hydralazine, etc. Metals: • thallium • arsenic • mercury
Immune mediated	Acute/chronic inflammatory demyelinating Associated with: • paraproteinaemia • cryoglobinaemia • acquired amyloidosis • Paraneoplastic
Hereditary	Hereditary sensory and autonomic neuropathy (type 1) Fabry's disease
Idiopathic	

Table 6.4 Pathological causes of asymmetrical painful neuropathies and neuropathic pain

Mononeuritis/mononeuritis multiplex	Diabetic: • cranial neuropathy • trunk/limb mononeuropathy • amyotrophy Vasculitic: • systemic of vasa nervorum: • polyarteritis nodosa • churg-Strauss syndrome • rheumatoid arthritis • lupus erythematosus • systemic sclerosis • wegener's granulomatosis • isolated angiitis of peripheral nerves Infectious/para-infectious: • HIV related • borreliosis • herpes zoster
Physical injury	Nerve entrapment: • carpal tunnel and other nerve compression • root compression (intervertebral disk herniation) • neuroma (post-traumatic, post-surgical, post-amputation Radiation induced Post-traumatic plexus neuropathy Tumour infiltration Phantom limb pain
Idiopathic neuritis	Brachial neuritis Lumbosacral neuritis
Cranial neuralgias	Trigeminal neuralgia Glossopharyngeal neuralgia

6.3 Well-recognized causes of peripheral neuropathic pain

6.3.1 Diabetic neuropathy

This is the most common cause of neuropathy in the Western world, affecting about 50% of diabetic patients over time. It is usually seen in diabetics over 50 years old, and is related directly to the toxic effects of hyperglycaemia. More recently, impaired glucose tolerance (pre-diabetes) has also been shown to be associated with painful peripheral neuropathy.

The most common form of neuropathy in diabetes mellitus is a distal symmetrical polyneuropathy, which is predominantly sensory. The main complaint is persistent distressing numbness and tingling, worse at night, often confined to the feet and lower legs. A deep aching may develop, with lancinating pain and burning. There is initial distal reduction in light touch, pain, and vibration sensation, but as the neuropathy progresses this extends more proximally and may involve the hands and trunk. Ankle jerks are reduced and mild weakness may occur. Painless foot ulceration together with autonomic neuropathy develops in severe cases with universal severe dysfunction of all nerve fibre populations due to demyelination with or without axonal degeneration. The upper limbs may also be involved.

Rarely, an acute painful diabetic neuropathy can present with profound weight loss and burning pain that is worse at night. This can follow an episode of ketosis or establishment of tight glycaemic control. There is little sensory or motor loss, but there is hyperalgesia and contact with clothing and bedding is unpleasant. Symptoms tend to improve with weight gain and adequate diabetic control. Occasionally, paraesthesiae and pain follow the institution of insulin therapy, but this tends to improve slowly with glycaemic control.

Painful asymmetric neuropathy, probably due to a vasculitis affecting small epineural vessels, is sometimes seen in older patients with mild or undetected diabetes. Pain often starts in the back or hip and spreads down the leg on one side. There is usually weakness and wasting of the pelvic girdle and thigh muscles. Recovery is normal, but may be incomplete. Acute diabetic mononeuropathy may result from infarction of a nerve.

Diabetic thoracolumbar radiculopathy due to a lesion proximal in the nerve root occurs in older patients with long-standing diabetes and may be associated with weight loss. It presents with girdle pain around the trunk, either unilateral or bilateral, and there may be abdominal wall weakness, cutaneous hyperaesthesia, or superficial sensory loss over the affected area. EMG changes can be detected in paraspinal and abdominal wall muscles. Recovery may be protracted, but ultimate prognosis is good.

6.3.2 **Post-herpetic neuralgia**

Shingles (herpes zoster infection) is frequently painful. Pain may persist in the affected area for more than 12 weeks following the healing of the herpetic skin lesions, especially in the elderly (50% of patients over 50 years old), to become post-herpetic neuralgia. It can be severe and debilitating, and may abate after months or continue for years.

Both peripheral and central mechanisms are involved. Minimal sensory loss characteristically produces abnormal sensitization of unmyelinated cutaneous nociceptors. Small-fibre deafferentation may profoundly impair pain and temperature sensation, giving allodynia to a moving stimulus (dynamic allodynia), almost certainly due to the formation of new connections between non-nociceptive large-diameter primary afferents and central pain transmission neurons. Deafferentation with loss of both large- and small-diameter fibres will give increased spontaneous activity in deafferented central neurons with or without reorganization of central connections, and severe spontaneous pain with hyperalgesia or allodynia. Each of these changes may be present to different degrees in any patient.

6.3.3 Trigeminal neuralgia

Trigeminal neuralgia is a sudden, usually unilateral, severe, brief, stabbing, recurrent pain in the distribution of one or more branches of the fifth cranial nerve. Eighty per cent (80%) of cases are idiopathic, and 66% of these have vascular pressure at the root entry zone. Other causes include demyelinating plaques in multiple sclerosis, angioma, brainstem infarcts, and tumours such as acoustic neuromas.

6.3.4 Post-surgical neuropathic pain

Post-surgical neuropathic pain can result from surgical section with deafferentation, compression, stretching, ischaemia, and infection of the nerve. It has been estimated that 10% of all surgery produces post-surgical neuropathic pain, including painful scars. During the process of regeneration of nerves, the axonal sprouts generate neural activity, which is most marked when neuromata develop. The consequent barrage of activity into the spinal cord leads to central sensitization.

6.3.5 Phantom limb pain

From very early childhood virtually everyone who has an amputation experiences sensations apparently arising from the amputated limb or organ. As time passes the phantom limb becomes less vivid, and the limb appears to telescope into the amputation stump, although most feel the phantom for the rest of their lives. Phantom limb pain is common, 80% of amputees having troublesome pain for at least one week every year, and many for considerably more of the year. The pain is frequently exacerbated by irritation in the stump, exhaustion, back pain, stress, or external factors such as changes in humidity.

6.3.6 Post-traumatic neuropathic pain

Traumatic lesions, such as brachial plexus avulsion from the spinal cord, frequently produce an intractable, persistent, severe, disabling pain that is a constant crushing and intermittent shooting pain.

6.3.7 Human immunodeficiency virus (HIV)

Various types of peripheral neuropathy may complicate HIV infection, producing pain in 30% of patients with HIV, the most common being a distal symmetrical polyneuropathy as a direct result of the infection. HIV-1 is highly neurotrophic and is present in the central nervous system in the earliest stages of infection, well before significant immunosuppression. Neuropathy can occur from the antiretroviral drugs, vitamin B_{12} deficiency associated with HIV, and concurrent alcoholism. Painful mononeuropathy multiplex related to focal vasculitis, or subacute cauda equina syndrome, or radiculopathy due to cytomegalovirus infection also occurs. Inflammatory demyelinating neuropathies may produce Guillain-Barré syndrome. Clearly, antiretroviral treatment may be helpful.

6.3.8 Nerve compression and entrapment neuropathies

A nerve may be mechanically constricted in a fibro-osseous tunnel or deformed by a fibrous band. Symptoms come on gradually (sensory more than motor, except in the elderly) and fluctuate with activity and rest. Systemic conditions should always be excluded that can make nerves prone to compression, such as diabetes, hypothyroidism, pregnancy, and amyloid, and hereditary liability to pressure palsies. Common sites are shown in Box 6.1.

6.3.9 Complex regional pain syndrome

Complex regional pain syndrome (CRPS) is associated with trauma, either mild with no nerve injury (type 1), or more major with nerve injury (type 2). Allodynia, hyperpathia, and autonomic signs are present. Autonomic changes are significant (see Chapter 8).

> **Box 6.1 Common sites for entrapment neuropathies**
>
> - Median nerve compression at wrist
> - Ulnar nerve in cubital canal at the elbow or in Guyon's canal at the wrist
> - Suprascapular nerve at spinoglenoid notch
> - Posterior interosseous nerve in the radial tunnel
> - Lateral femoral cutaneous nerve of the thigh (meralgia paraesthetica) at the inguinal ligament
> - Obturator nerve in the obturator canal
> - Posterior tibial nerve in the tarsal tunnel
> - Interdigital plantar nerve (Morton's metatarsalgia) in the plantar fascia between the heads of the third and fourth metatarsals.

6.3.10 **Cancer**

Neuropathic pain can occur in cancer, frequently due to tumour invasion, but also because of radiation fibrosis, radiation myelopathy, chemotherapy, or surgery (especially after mastectomy or thoraco-tomy). If standard analgesic, adjunctive, and neuropathic drug therapy is inadequate, then interventions can be useful, such as spinal drug delivery systems, or neurodestructive techniques such as intrathecal neurolysis or percutaneous cordotomy. Paraneoplastic neuropathies occur as remote effects of carcinoma and can precede detection of malignancy by months or years (see Chapter 9).

6.4 **Less well-recognized causes**

6.4.1 **Guillain-Barré syndrome**

Acute inflammatory neuropathies can affect cranial, respiratory, and upper limbs early in the course of the disease, generally as an au-toimmune response. Guillain-Barré syndrome, a demyelinating poly-neuropathy, may have an autoimmune base following an infection, and affects peripheral nerves predominantly, concentrating on the region where the anterior and posterior spinal roots fuse. It is always bilateral but not always symmetrical, and produces motor paralysis or weakness and sensory deficit. Generally recovery occurs. Pain, paraesthesiae, and dysaesthesiae commonly occur, although motor abnormalities predominate.

6.4.2 **Other autoimmune neuropathies**

Polyarteritis nodosa, Churg-Strauss syndrome, rheumatoid arthritis, lupus erythematosus, systemic sclerosis, and Wegener's granuloma-tosis can produce a vasculitic neuropathy, usually a mononeuritis multiplex. Cryoglobulinaemia may produce a mononeuritis multiplex or symmetrical polyneuropathy with painful dysaesthesiae. Primary amyloidosis presents with painful dysaesthesiae and numbness, with disturbance of small-fibre activity in pain, temperature, and autonom-ic small-fibres.

Neuralgic amyotrophy may develop suddenly in an otherwise healthy individual or follow an infection, surgical procedure, child-birth, or an injection of vaccine or antibiotic to produce a brachial neuralgia. It usually begins with a severe pain around the shoulder on one side, followed rapidly by profound weakness and atrophy, usually of the C5 and C6 myotomes. Movement of the involved muscles exacerbates the pain. Pain usually settles in a few days or weeks, and recovery is normally good.

6.4.3 **Hypothyroid neuropathy**

There is a high incidence of carpal tunnel syndrome in hypothyroid-ism, but a sensorimotor polyneuropathy can also occur with painful dysaesthesiae and lancinating pains in the hands and feet, and glove and stocking sensory loss, with occasional distal weakness and wasting. It improves with levothyroxine (thyroxine) replacement therapy.

6.4.4 Deficiency states

Neuropathy due to nutritional deficiency is uncommon in the developed world, and is usually seen in association with alcoholism, malabsorption, gastrointestinal surgery to produce weight loss in obesity, and prolonged stay in intensive care units. The common deficiency states are vitamins B_1 (thiamine), B_6 (pyridoxine) (associated with antituberculous treatment with isoniazid, and antihypertensive treatment with hydralazine), and niacin. Extremely high doses of pyridoxine may also cause a neuropathy. Alcoholic neuropathy is considered to be due to vitamin B_1 deficiency, and symptoms are non-specific.

6.4.5 Toxic neuropathies

Arsenic ingestion will produce a systemic illness (gastrointestinal symptoms, anaemia, jaundice, hyperkeratosis of palms and soles, and later white transverse banding of nails), with associated neuropathy and aching or burning pain, tingling, or numbness in the fingers and toes spreading proximally.

Thallium ingestion will produce a rapidly progressing painful sensory neuropathy, whereas mercury will affect the central nervous system (visual field defects, ataxia, mental impairment), but a polyneuropathy can develop early with distal paraesthesiae that may involve the tongue.

Peripheral neuropathy is the significant dose-limiting side-effect of many cytotoxic and antiretroviral drugs. Ten per cent (10%) of patients on zalcitabine or stavudine have to discontinue therapy with the development of neuropathy.

6.4.6 Hereditary neuropathies

Hereditary sensory and autonomic neuropathy (HSAN) type 1, an autosomal dominant inherited condition, can produce spontaneous burning, aching, or lancinating pain. Fabry's disease may also present with burning sensations in the hands and lower legs, with tender legs in young boys or men, and pain so severe that walking is limited.

6.5 Treatment options

6.5.1 Analgesics

Frequently, neuropathic pain responds poorly to standard analgesics. Tricyclic antidepressants have useful efficacy, but their side-effects are problematic. Antiepileptic drugs have similar efficacy and can be used with tricyclics or in combination with different antiepileptics (see Chapter 11). Capsaicin cream is useful for allodynia. Opioids can be useful, especially in severe pain, and both tramadol and oxycodone have been shown to be useful in diabetic neuropathy (see Chapter 14).

6.5.2 Non-drug options

Neuromodulation using TENS, acupuncture, or spinal cord stimulation can also be helpful (see Chapters 16 and 17). TENS electrodes need to be applied over accessible functioning nerves proximal to the lesion, or over the painful area (which is usually too large to be practical) that has normal sensation. Acupuncture is not practical in the long term.

Trigeminal neuralgia, or other nerve compression problems, can respond well to decompression surgery, and trigeminal neuralgia can also be helped by per-foraminal ovale neurodestructive procedures. Neuropathic cancer pain can also respond to interventions such as spinal drug delivery systems or, if unilateral, percutaneous cordotomy can be invaluable.

Key references

Fields, H.L., Rowbotham, M., Baron, R. (1998). Postherpetic neuralgia: irritable nociceptors and deafferentation. *Neurobiol. Disease*, **5**, 209–27.

Grady, K.M., Severn, A.M., Eldridge, P.R. (2002). *Key topics in chronic pain* (2nd edn). Taylor & Francis, Abingdon.

Jensen, T.S. and Gottrup, H. (2003). Assessment of neuropathic pain. In: T.S. Jensen, P.R. Wilson, and A.S.C. Rice (ed.) *Clinical pain management: chronic pain,* pp. 113–24. Arnold, London.

Shembalkar, P. and Anand, P. (2003). Peripheral neuropathies. In: T.S. Jensen, P.R. Wilson, and A.S.C. Rice (ed.) *Clinical pain management: chronic pain,* pp. 355–66. Arnold, London.

Smith AG, Singleton JR. (2008) Impaired glucose tolerance and neuropathy. *Neurologist,* **14**(1), 23–9.

Sternbach, R.A. (1963). Congenital insensitivity to pain: a critique. *Psychol Bull,* **60**, 252–64.

Chapter 7

Central neuropathic pain

David Bowsher

> **Key points**
>
> - Central neuropathic pain can arise following damage to spinothalamocortical pathways in the spinal cord and brain
> - Stroke, multiple sclerosis, and spinal cord injury (trauma or disease) are the predominant causes
> - Central neuropathic pain is wrongly considered a rarity; several tens of thousands of cases exist in the UK and it can develop up to two years after stroke
> - Tactile and cold allodynia are common
> - Central neuropathic pain seems to be less responsive to co-analgesics and opioids than peripheral neuropathic pain though novel methods of pain control are being developed; some show promise.

7.1 Background

Most health professionals, on seeing the phrase 'central neuropathic pain', think immediately of central post-stroke pain (CPSP), or as it erroneously used to be called, thalamic syndrome. In fact, central neuropathic pain (CNP) occurs after a number of other central nervous system insults. High on the list are spinal cord injury (SCI) and syringomyelia, as well as some other supraspinal conditions such as Wallenberg's syndrome and multiple sclerosis. Central neuropathic pain has been defined as pain arising from damage to the ascending spinothalamocortical pathways, their relays, or end-stations in the spinal cord or brain. This seems to the present author to be the best and most comprehensive definition of CNP. Furthermore, CNP shares with peripheral neuropathic pains the useful clinical definition of 'pain in an area of altered sensation'.

7.2 Epidemiology of central neuropathic pain

7.2.1 Stroke and spinal cord injury

Central post-stroke pain is the form of CNP with which most pain practitioners are most frequently concerned. CPSP was originally called 'thalamic syndrome' because the first cases described 100 years ago had lesions in the thalamus, or more precisely, in the post-erolateroventral thalamic nucleus, and so the name 'thalamic syndrome' became sanctified. Leaving aside the large number of cerebral stroke lesions outside the thalamus which are now known to cause CPSP, it has more recently been shown that only 25% of patients with classical (posterolateroventral thalamic) lesions develop CPSP (Figure 7.1).

Figure 7.1 Central post-stroke pain (CPSP) patient with thalamic lesion (arrowed) on left. *Clinical features*: right-sided burning pain, raised tactile (von Frey), warm, cool, and hot pain thresholds; mechanical pain threshold (skin-fold pinch) not raised. No allodynia.

There are about 100,000 strokes per year in the UK and one-third of these are fatal. Of the rest, the incidence of CPSP is about 8–10,000 cases per year. Since most cases of CPSP are in patients who do not have very severe motor deficits, the patients tend to have quite a good survival rate, so that the prevalence of CPSP in the UK is probably of the order of 50,000. In the USA, these figures may be multiplied by five, so that there may be a quarter of a million CPSP sufferers.

CNP probably affects two-thirds of patients with SCI. The prevalence of SCI is not accurately recorded, but there are of course a large number of cases, caused not only by extreme sports but in the main by traffic accidents. Similarly, around 30% of patients with multiple sclerosis develop CNP, though the exact prevalence is hard to determine.

7.2.2 **CNP in the population**

Given the very large numbers of patients with CNP (tens of thousands of cases in the UK and hundreds of thousands in North America), it remains a matter of mystery as to why CNP is regarded as a rarity by health professionals. The fact that it has multiple causes may contribute to this notion, and possibly interfere intellectually with its treatment as an entity.

It has already been stated that one-third of patients with spinal cord injuries do not have CNP. While figures for other forms of CNP are not so well established, the failure to develop neuropathic pain in a large number of subjects with many forms of damage to the peripheral or central nervous system is perhaps what should really be occupying our attention when seeking a pathophysiological explanation for the condition.

7.3 **Features of central neuropathic pain**

7.3.1 **Pain**

This may be permanent or intermittent, constant or fluctuating in intensity. Descriptions vary according to the individual patient, and of course to the language and culture group to which the patient belongs. Textbooks and teachers are very fond of saying that the pain is characteristically 'burning', but this is because other pains are not so described – not more than 50% of CNP patients use the word 'burning'. The pain may be aching or throbbing, stabbing or lancinating, like many non-neuropathic pains. The nearest most healthy people get to it is sunburn, which is a *temporary* neuropathic pain due to reversible nerve damage, or to holding a snowball in the hand for too long—'ice-burn'.

Nearly half of stroke patients who have CNP feel pain on regaining consciousness, and 60% develop the pain within three months.

However, the rest take up to 2 years to develop pain. This means that a large proportion of CNP patients will have been discharged from specialized care by the time they develop CNP. Family practitioners and nurses should therefore be on the lookout for late-developing CNP in stroke patients. CNP onset following SCI is also not immediate in many cases.

7.3.2 Altered sensation

The painful area always occurs *within* (i.e. is smaller than) an area of altered superficial skin sensation. The sensations most frequently changed (i.e. with raised thresholds) are innocuous and noxious temperature sensations, sharpness, and mechanical pain. That is, the sensations subserved by smaller peripheral nerve fibres are the most affected. Pain intensity seems to correlate in particular with the degree of innocuous temperature deficit. Tactile and vibratory sensations are less frequently affected.

Testing for innocuous changes

Raised thresholds for innocuous temperature means inability to appreciate warmth in something slightly warmer than the patient's skin, such as the examiner's finger; or slightly cooler, such as a metal spoon or tuning fork. It does not mean near-boiling or iced water in a test-tube. Similarly, sharpness does not mean shoving a pin or needle deep into the tissues and twisting it— that's painful! Sharpness is tested by seeing whether the patient, with eyes closed, can tell the difference between the head and the point of a pin gently applied to the skin surface.

Testing for mechanical and thermal pain

Mechanical pain can be tested by grasping and squeezing a skin fold between finger and thumb, and heat pain with a test-tube containing water (or any other object) at 50–60°. It is very important to specify whether mechanical or thermal pain is affected; there is no such thing as 'pain' (unspecified), nor of course is there such a thing as 'painful stimulation'. *Noxious* (potentially tissue-damaging) stimulation, either mechanical or thermal, *would* result in a sensation of pain in a normal intact person, but not in the unconscious person or a patient with lost sensation in the stimulated area.

Heat and mechanical pains are in different categories from the periphery onwards. This is illustrated in the periphery by the fact that application of capsaicin abolishes response to painful or noxious heat, but not to painful or noxious mechanical stimulation. The differentiation is maintained within the central nervous system, as shown by the fact that some central lesions interfere with appreciation of stimuli of one noxious type but not the other.

Since Nature conveniently provides a control in all cases, responses to sensory tests should be compared between the affected area and the mirror-image unaffected area on the other side.

Figure 7.2 Pontine lesion. Lesion in pons (arrowed), just below fourth ventricle, above which is the cerebellum. ***Clinical features***: throbbing pain in left side, tactile (von Frey) threshold unaffected; mechanical pain threshold (skin-fold pinch) raised; warm and cool thresholds minimally (perhaps non-significantly) raised; hot pain threshold significantly raised. No allodynia.

7.3.3 Allodynia

This is defined as pain experienced on stimulation by a non-noxious stimulus. Allodynia usually occurs within the painful area, and is encountered in about 70% of patients with CPSP. The commonest form is tactile allodynia, which is elicited by light brushing and occurs in 50% of cases. Less common are cold allodynia, elicited by non-noxious cold stimulation, and movement allodynia, elicited by active or passive stretching of muscles or tendons. Unlike the sensations whose thresholds are most frequently raised, the sensations most frequently causing allodynia are those subserved by large peripheral nerve fibres, thus demonstrating the important interactions between afferent fibres of different sizes at the first or subsequent synapses within the central nervous system. More than one form of allodynia may occur in the same patient.

61

Just occasionally, allodynia within the painful area can be elicited by appropriate stimulation at some distant body site, but always on the same side as the CNP pain. Patients usually volunteer this recondite information (e.g. 'My chest hurts every time I brush the side of my calf') because it's so unusual, unexpected, and inexplicable.

7.3.4 Autonomic component

When large body areas are involved, such as a whole limb in CPSP, the affected area may feel cold, both subjectively and objectively. This is evidence of an autonomic component to CNP. The coldness (vasoconstriction) can be got rid of by prescribing a calcium-channel blocker, but as this doesn't relieve the pain, it's not worth doing unless the cold sensation in itself really disturbs the patient.

7.3.5 Site of the lesion

The intellectual challenge of locating the site of the lesion has been removed by the universality of imaging. But for those who wish to use imaging as confirmation of their diagnosis, the following may be borne in mind with regard to CNP:

• *history* — ?stroke; ?injury; ?sudden or gradual onset
• *distribution of pain and sensory change* — there should be no difficulty in distinguishing infra- from supraspinal causes of CNP. In supraspinal CNP, lesions above the decussation of the medial lemniscus in the upper medulla oblongata give rise to both pain and sensory loss on the contralateral side. Low medullary lesions, however, cause loss of soft touch sensation in the ipsilateral face but pain and temperature loss in the contralateral limb(s): Wallenberg's syndrome.

In cases where all symptoms occur on the side opposite the lesion, if the greatest pain and/or deficit occurs in the extremities, the lesion is most probably in the thalamus or cortex; but if the greatest pain or deficit is not in the extremities, the lesion is probably infrathalamic. If the most severe pain is in the face, the lesion is probably infratentorial.

7.4 Possible mechanisms of CNP

It had earlier been suggested that one mechanism of CNP might lie in the level of particular, but unknown, transmitters and/or receptors in the central nervous system. Thus if certain transmitters or receptors are depleted as a result of insult to the central nervous system, CNP might ensue. A similar suggestion with regard to pain following SCI has also been made. If the depletion is sudden and massive, immediate pain occurs; if gradual, pain develops gradually. If levels of transmitters or receptors are up-regulated by treatment or by Nature, recovery takes place. This hypothesis is supported by a number of investigations involving specific receptors, such as NK_1 serotonin receptors, spinal $5HT_3$ receptors, or transmitters such as ubiquitin C-terminal hydrolase. However, it should be noted that the above hypothesis does not explain why CNP is sometimes relieved by the occurrence of a further stroke, resulting in yet more damage to the brain.

7.5 Treatment

7.5.1 Co-analgesics

Up to about the 1970s, CNP was mainly treated by the administration of larger and larger doses of stronger and stronger analgesics, including morphine and diamorphine (heroin). The unfortunate result of this was the existence of a large number of agonized junkies. In the 1960s, it was found that trigeminal neuralgia (now known not to be a typical form of neuropathic pain) could be relieved by carbamazepine and subsequently other antiepileptics. Thus began the treatment of CNP with a mixture of analgesics and antiepileptics, resulting in overweight, cognitively challenged patients.

Alongside this, however, it had been found that tricyclic antidepressants of the amitriptyline group, which had noradrenergic as well as serotonergic properties, were effective in the treatment of neuropathic pain of peripheral origin, particularly post-herpetic neuralgia. This finding was applied with some success to the treatment of CPSP, in which it was found, as in post-herpetic neuralgia, that the sooner after pain onset such treatment was initiated, the greater the possibility of success. If treatment was commenced within six months of pain onset, almost 90% were relieved; and within 12 months, two-thirds; subsequent to this, the proportion fell to less than half.

Ami- and nortriptyline, which often have undesirable side-effects, are noradrenergic and serotonergic. Pure serotonergic antidepressants, such as fluoxetine, although having many fewer adverse effects, are unfortunately virtually useless in the treatment of CNP.

However, the idea of effective antiepileptic treatment, despite the failure of carbamazepine, continued to haunt many physicians; and modern antiepileptics such as gabapentin and pregabalin, together with lamotrigine, have been found to produce pain relief in a proportion of cases.

7.5.2 Other approaches

Modern pharmacotherapy has re-evaluated opioid treatment in a much more careful way. A number of judiciously applied opioids, such as oxycodone, or a mixture of dextromethorphan and morphine, have been successfully deployed in a proportion of cases. Membrane-stabilizing drugs, such as mexiletine, have been shown to be useful in the treatment of cases not responding to tricyclics.

In our series of over 100 cases of CPSP treated by non-opioid pharmacotherapy, about half achieved total or substantial relief of their pain. In intractable cases (of which, sadly, there are far too many), a number of interventional techniques have been, and are being, tried. For instance, electrical stimulation of the spinal cord or brain has met with a certain degree of success.

It is to be hoped that a better understanding of the molecular mechanisms of CNP will lead to more rational and effective treatment.

Key references

Beric, A., Dimitrijevic, M.R., Lindblom, U. (1988). Central dysesthesia syndrome in spinal cord injury patients. *Pain*, **34**, 109–16.

Bogousslavsky, J., Regli, F., Uske, A. (1988). Thalamic infarcts: clinical syndromes, etiology, and prognosis. *Neurology*, **38**, 837–48.

Boivie, J. (2006). Central Pain. In: McMahon, S.B., and Koltzenburg, M. (ed.) *Wall & Melzack's Textbook of Pain*, 5th edn., **67**, 1057–74. Elsevier Churchill Livingstone.

Bowsher, D. (1996). Central Pain: Clinical and Physiological Characteristics. *J. Neurol. Neurosurg. Psychiat.*, **61**, 62–9.

Bowsher, D., Leijon, G., and Thuomas, K-A. (1988). Central Post-Stroke Pain: Correlation of Magnetic Resonance Imaging with Clinical Pain Characteristics and Sensory Abnormalities. *Neurology*, **51**, 1352–8.

Bowsher, D. (2005). Allodynia in relation to lesion site in central post-stroke pain. *J. Pain*, **6**, 736–40.

Cassinari, V., Pagni, C.A. (1969). *Central Pain: A Neurosurgical Survey*. Harvard University Press, Cambridge, MA.

Dejerine, J., Roussy, J. (1906). Le syndrome thalamique. *Rev Neurol*, **14**, 521–32.

Ramachandran V.S., McGeoch P.D., Williams L., Arcilla G. (2007). Rapid relief of thalamic pain syndrome by vestibular caloric stimulation. Neurocase; **13**: 185–8.

Chapter 8

Complex regional pain syndrome

Dudley Bush

Key points

- Complex regional pain syndrome is the current name for the conditions previously called reflex sympathetic dystrophy (now CRPS type I) and causalgia (now CRPS type II).
- It occurs in distal limbs following trauma or surgery, is not related to intensity of initial insult, and is idiopathic in 10% of cases. There are around 10,000 cases in the UK and it is four times more common in females.
- Mechanisms underlying CRPS are complex but may involve neurogenic inflammation.
- Weakness and autonomic changes commonly accompany pain.
- Treatment is based on relief of pain (with co-analgesics, opioids, and neuromodulation) combined with restoration of function, so early referral and treatment is essential to prevent irreversible trophic changes and contractures.

8.1 Background

8.1.1 Clinical definitions

Complex regional pain syndrome (CRPS) is the current name for an uncommon condition in which severe spontaneous or evoked pain persists disproportionate to an initiating event. CRPS commonly occurs in the distal limb following trauma or surgery, but can occur spontaneously in any body part and is not related to the severity of the initiating noxious insult. There are usually accompanying features including altered sensation, swelling, vasomotor instability, motor abnormality, and osteoporosis. Originally described in relation to traumatic nerve injury by Weir Mitchell during the American Civil War, and later by Sudeck in 1900 after wrist fracture, the condition has been recognized for many years but has only recently been systematically classified and studied. Previous names include reflex sympathetic dystrophy (RSD), sympathetically maintained pain, algodystrophy, Sudeck's atrophy, and causalgia.

The clinical term CRPS was suggested in 1994 by the International Association for the Study of Pain (IASP) in an attempt to improve recognition and diagnosis of the condition (Box 8.1). It was hoped that the previous overemphasis upon involvement of the sympathetic nervous system in diagnosis would be avoided and that the confusion in nomenclature would be reduced. Type II CRPS is similar to type I except that initiating trauma must involve nerve injury. It is important that all the features are present, not just pain.

8.1.2 Epidemiology

In a US population, the incidence of CRPS has been found to be approximately five per 100,000 years at risk, with a prevalence of 21 per 100,000, and a female:male ratio of 4:1. Half of all cases follow trauma, more commonly of the upper limb, with rates of 7% to 37% following wrist fracture. Limb surgery is a common cause; estimates of incidence are 2–4% after arthroscopic knee surgery, 2–5% after carpal tunnel surgery, 13% after ankle surgery, and 1–13% after total knee arthroplasty. CRPS may occur in other locations or follow other initiating events, including myocardial infarction and stroke, and in 10% of cases no precipitating event can be identified.

8.2 Clinical features

8.2.1 Sensory disturbance

Pain and hyperalgesia (increased response to a nociceptive stimulus) are the main features of CRPS, with the majority of patients reporting pain at rest. Common pain descriptors are burning, aching, and shooting. Allodynia (pain upon light touch) is a common feature in CRPS and hypo-aesthesia (decreased sensitivity) is common.

Box 8.1 Clinical definition of complex regional pain syndrome

- Presence of an initiating noxious event or cause of immobilization
- type I—without obvious nerve injury
- type II—with obvious nerve injury
- Continuing pain, allodynia, or hyperalgesia disproportionate to the initiating event and not limited to a single nerve territory
- Evidence at some time of oedema, changes in skin blood flow, or abnormal sudomotor activity or motor symptoms.
- Other diagnoses are excluded, for example missed fracture, connective tissue disease

Mechanical allodynia is reported by most CRPS patients and manifests as pain upon movement. The sensory changes often do not occur in a neuroanatomical distribution and can become widespread.

8.2.2 Motor disturbance

Weakness is very common in CRPS, initially because of pain-dependent guarding, but later tremor, myoclonus, and focal dystonia are seen. Many patients have exaggerated deep tendon reflexes on the affected side. Later the limb is neglected and patients are often observed to ignore a functionless hand held on their lap which is devoid of any spontaneous movement. Most patients have significant motor involvement.

8.2.3 Autonomic disturbance

In the acute stage of CRPS there is usually distal oedema in the affected limb and the skin is warm, red, and glossy. Some months later the limb becomes cold with mottled blue skin (Figure 8.1). These changes are due to changes in regulation of peripheral perfusion.

A minority of cases never exhibit the warm phase. The temperature difference between affected and normal limb is usually more than 2°C, although the magnitude and direction of this difference will vary according to environment. The specificity of the temperature change is high for diagnosis of CRPS, although sensitivity is only 32% under resting conditions. Sudomotor abnormality ranges from hyperhydrosis through to bone-dry skin.

Figure 8.1 Early features of CRPS—note swelling and dusky appearance in left hand

8.2.4 Trophic changes

In the initial stages of CRPS there is increased hair and nail growth, while later this situation reverses with loss of skin features including hair. Eventually muscle atrophy and fixed contractures can occur.

8.2.5 Natural history

Previously three sequential stages of CRPS were described: an early acute phase resembling inflammation, an intermediate dystrophic phase with more marked pain, sensory and motor changes, and a late atrophic stage, typified by loss of function, severe trophic features, and contracture. However, not all patients follow this progression and the existence of sequential phases of CRPS is no longer recognized as useful in the diagnosis or management of CRPS. Indeed, some patients exhibit decreased skin temperature from the outset; this form of CRPS is associated with a poor prognosis, including ulceration and infection sometimes requiring amputation.

There is proximal spread from the original area affected in a contiguous manner in most cases, while in 70% symptoms and signs may appear in independent non-contiguous sites. Rarely, symptoms and signs will appear in the opposite limb as a mirror image of the original.

8.3 Diagnosis

CRPS is primarily a clinical diagnosis and the condition is probably overdiagnosed. More robust diagnostic criteria with high specificity but lower sensitivity have been proposed for research purposes (Box 8.2). There is no confirmatory diagnostic test for CRPS although other differential diagnoses may need to be excluded with appropriate investigations. Among the most useful investigations to support the diagnosis of CRPS are:

- Plain radiology—osteoporotic change is common after the first few weeks
- Three-phase bone scintigram—a three-phase bone scan with Technetium-99m will show increased uptake in later stages of the condition
- MRI—this will show widespread oedema in deep connective tissue, muscle, and peri-articular tissue
- Thermography—this will demonstrate any temperature difference between affected and normal limbs.

> **Box 8.2 Research criteria for diagnosis of CRPS**
>
> - Continuing pain disproportionate to inciting event
> - At least one symptom from each of the following four categories:
>   - sensory (hyperasthesia)
>   - vasomotor (temperature asymmetry, skin colour change, or asymmetry)
>   - sudomotor (oedema, sweating change, or asymmetry)
>   - motor/trophic (reduced range of motion, weakness, tremor dystonia/nail, hair, skin changes)
> - Must display at least one sign in two or more of the following categories:
>   - sensory (hyperalgesia, allodynia)
>   - vasomotor (temperature asymmetry, skin colour change, or asymmetry)
>   - sudomotor (oedema, sweating change, or asymmetry)
>   - motor/trophic (reduced range of motion, weakness, tremor dystonia/nail, hair, skin changes).

8.4 Pathophysiology

8.4.1 Overview

It seems most likely that CRPS is a systemic disease involving both the central and peripheral nervous system in susceptible individuals. Recent research favours the central mechanisms as the most important in maintaining CRPS. The clinical course of CRPS is so variable that it is likely that there is no single mechanism involved and indeed there is some ongoing debate regarding the existence of CRPS as a single entity. Several mechanisms are thought to be relevant and are not necessarily specific to CRPS. The pathophysiology is clearly multifactorial and the exact nature of the initiating event may be relatively unimportant.

8.4.2 Regional or neurogenic inflammation

The acute stage of CRPS resembles acute inflammation although attempts to show typical products of inflammation in peripheral tissues produce inconsistent results. Primary nociceptive afferent activation by cytokines released following trauma results in retrograde release of neuropeptides in the periphery, including substance P and calcitonin gene-related peptide. This process of neurogenic inflammation may produce the inflammatory-like features of CRPS, including increased skin temperature, oedema, and the trophic changes.

8.4.3 Sympathetic nervous system

There is considerable evidence suggesting that the sympathetic nervous system has a role in chronic neuropathic inflammatory pain states (Box 8.3). Following the initial skin temperature increase due to neurogenic inflammation, there is evidence of central sympathetic dysfunction manifest as limb temperature decrease with increased sweating. Initially, sympathetic noradrenergic control of blood vessels is reduced, producing vasodilation, and subsequently it is thought that the denervated blood vessels develop an increased sensitivity to catecholamine, resulting in vasoconstriction. There may be additional central failure of sympathetic control of vasoconstriction. There is evidence that in CRPS functional adrenoceptors are expressed on primary nociceptive afferents because subcutaneous injection of noradrenaline (norepinephrine) is painful while sympathetic blockade relieves pain.

The exact role of the sympathetic nervous system in CRPS remains controversial and it seems likely that pain due to sympathetic dysfunction—termed 'sympathetically maintained pain' (SMP)—overlaps with CRPS but is also relevant in other types neuropathic pain, while in many cases of CRPS, SMP is not relevant.

8.4.4 Central neuroplasticity

Patients with CRPS often report numbness and hyperalgesia in a neurological distribution outside that of the original injury, sometimes extending to a hemisensory impairment. These changes reverse if CRPS pain is relieved. This implies central nervous system plasticity at spinal or supraspinal level and there is evidence for both from studies using positron emission tomography and magnetoencephalography (MEG). MEG studies have demonstrated cortical reorganization of hand representation in patients with CRPS, which reverses with effective analgesia (Figure 8.2) (see Chapter 2). Similar changes in cortical representation are observed in other neuropathic pain conditions, for example phantom limb pain. Such central changes are assuming increasing importance in the understanding of the pathophysiology of CRPS.

Box 8.3 Supportive evidence for sympathetic system involvement in chronic neuropathic pain

- Increase in number of adrenoceptors in skin
- Expression of adrenoceptors in peripheral sensory afferents
- Topical α_2-adrenoceptor agonists decrease pain in the affected region (by pre-synaptic decrease in noradrenaline (norepinephrine) release)
- Sympathectomy reduces pain in some cases
- Stress or sympathetic stimulation increases pain.

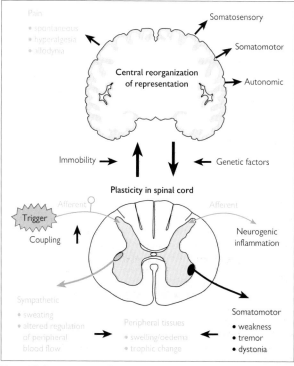

Figure 8.2 Sensory, motor and autonomic changes in CRPS type I. Changes are triggered by nociceptive afferent input. Afferent neurons may become sensitized to catecholamine by receptor expression or coupling to sympathetic efferents. CRPS is maintained by reorganization within the spinal cord resulting in retrograde neurogenic inflammation. Reorganization in higher centres results in pain, motor changes, and modified autonomic output.

8.4.5 Immobility

There is experimental evidence that prolonged immobilization can lead to changes similar to CRPS without the need for an injury or noxious event. The magnitude of the changes from such experimental immobilization is less than in clinical CRPS, suggesting that this mechanism is only contributory.

8.4.6 Genetic factors

An association with HLA-DR13 and HLA-DQ1 in patients with CRPS has been reported, suggesting a genetic susceptibility to CRPS. This might explain why only a few patients subject to a given trauma go on to develop CRPS.

8.4.7 Psychological factors

No specific psychological factors have been identified that predispose to CRPS, although secondary depression is common.

8.5 Treatment

There is no specific treatment for CRPS, perhaps because of the limited understanding of the underlying mechanisms. The management aims of type I and type II CRPS are similar and focus on the relief of pain and the restoration of function. There is very little good quality evidence to guide specific management of CRPS, a recent review identifying only 12 high quality studies.

8.5.1 Physical therapy

It is suggested that restoration of function to the affected limb reduces pain and improves prognosis and this remains the cornerstone of current treatment. Physiotherapy is the standard initial treatment for CRPS, using progressive desensitization and mobilization techniques, although progress may be limited by severe pain requiring additional treatment. It is important that active physical therapy is used and not the passive movement of an anaesthetized limb.

More specialized techniques have been used in CRPS, such as motor imagery training. This consists of sequential periods of hand laterality recognition, imagined movements, and lastly mirror movements. This technique has been shown to improve the symptoms of CRPS compared to passive mobilization. It is thought that the active nature of the treatment corrects inappropriate cortical remapping and thus it might be considered a mechanism-based treatment approach.

8.5.2 Medication

Non-steroidal anti-inflammatory drugs, opioids, and most co-analgesics have been used in the management of CRPS, using standard principles for neuropathic pain, with variable success and limited supportive evidence. The oral route is usual although occasionally opioids and co-analgesics, especially the α_2 adrenergic antagonist clonidine, are delivered intrathecally (unlicensed use). There is evidence that systemic steroid, biphosphonates and calcitonin are modestly effective in CRPS of less than six months duration.

8.5.3 Sympathetic nervous system blockade

Sympathetic interventions have been a traditional treatment for RSD for several decades because of early reports of efficacy. The sympathetic nervous system may be inhibited peripherally by means of intravenous regional sympathetic blockade comprising the injection of guanethidine (or bretylium; however this may not be readily available) and local anaesthetic distal to a limb tourniquet. The guanethidine acts by temporarily displacing noradrenaline (norepinephrine) from adrenergic nerve endings. More proximal sympathetic blockade can be achieved with thoracic sympathectomy or stellate ganglion block for the upper limb and lumbar sympathectomy for the lower limb, temporarily using local anaesthetic or more permanently with neurolytic agents. Recently there has been an appreciation that sympathetic blockade is useful in only a minority of patients with CRPS.

8.5.4 Somatic nerve blocks

Somatic local anaesthetic nerve blocks are used to facilitate physiotherapy and rehabilitation in CRPS by providing pain relief. Although there are no controlled trials there are numerous reports of continuous peripheral nerve blocks having been used in the management of CRPS. Commonly used blocks include continuous brachial plexus block and lumbar plexus blockade.

8.5.5 Amputation

Amputation remains a therapeutic option in severe CRPS; it is rarely recommended by clinicians but is often suggested by patients. High-quality evidence of effectiveness is lacking and amputation is certainly not a guaranteed solution for CRPS. The risk of long-term complications, including persisting pain and phantom pain, is real.

8.5.6 Neuromodulation

Neuromodulation involves the modification of pain transmission using non-destructive methods, the most common being high-frequency electrical stimulation. Transcutaneous electrical nerve stimulation (TENS; see Chapter 16) is commonly employed in the early management of CRPS, although the evidence of effectiveness is equivocal. The more invasive and expensive option of spinal cord stimulation (SCS; see Chapter 17), using an implanted epidural electrode stimulating system, has been demonstrated to have a modest beneficial effect in CRPS when combined with physical therapy. Minor technical problems are relatively common and SCS is usually a late treatment option.

8.5.7 Free radical scavengers

The demonstration of peripheral inflammatory mediators in CRPS has resulted in the use of free radical scavengers in an attempt to reduce the tissue-damaging effects of inflammation. Topical dimethyl sulfoxide has been found to be effective for pain relief in warm CRPS, while systemic N-acetyl cysteine is effective in cold CRPS. Neither agent is in common use. Note these are unlicensed uses.

8.5.8 Prevention of CRPS following surgery

The development of CRPS as a complication of surgery is unpredictable and so prevention is difficult, but it is recommended to avoid surgery on a limb currently affected by CRPS to avoid aggravation of the symptoms. Regional anaesthetic techniques are suggested to reduce the incidence and recurrence of CRPS, especially if sympathetic blockade is achieved. The use of free radical scavengers and various adrenergic blockers, for example ketanserin, have been suggested but evidence of effectiveness is limited. In general, effective multimodal peri-operative analgesia is probably the most effective way to guard against the development of CRPS.

Key references

Birklein, F. (2005). Complex regional pain syndrome. *J Neurol*, **252**, 131–8.

Drummond P., Finch P. (2006) Sensory changes in the forehead of patients with complex regional pain syndrome. *Pain*, **123**, 83–9.

Harden N., Swan M., King A. (2006) Treatment of complex regional pain syndrome: functional restoration. *Clinical Journal of Pain*, **22**, 422–4.

Harden N., Bruehl S., Stanton-Hicks M. (2007) Proposed new diagnostic criteria for complex regional pain syndrome. *Pain Medicine*, **8**, 326–331

Janig, W. and Baron, R. (2003). Complex regional pain syndrome: mystery explained. *Lancet Neurology*, **2**, 687–91.

Ochoa, J.L. (1999). Truths, errors and lies around 'reflex sympathetic dystrophy' and complex regional pain syndrome. *J Neurol*, 246, 875–9.

Stanton-Hicks, M., Janig, W., Hassenbusch, S., Haddox, J.D., Boas, R., Wilson, P. (1995). Reflex sympathetic dystrophy: changing concepts and taxonomy. *Pain*, **63**, 127–33.

Taylor R., Van Buyten J.P., Buscher E. (2006) Spinal cord stimulation for complex regional pain syndrome. A systematic review of the clinical and cost effectiveness literature and assessment of prognostic factors. *European Journal of Pain*, **10**, 91–101.

Uceyler N. Eberle T. Rolke R. Birklein F. Sommer C. (2007) Differential expression patterns of cytokines in complex regional pain syndrome. *Pain*, **132**, 195–205.

Chapter 9

Cancer neuropathic pain

Fliss E. Murtagh and Irene J. Higginson

Key points

- Around a third of cancer pains may have a neuropathic component and mixed pathology is more usual than 'pure' neuropathic pain
- Compression and infiltration of nerves by tumour are the most common causes
- Treatment-induced damage (chemotherapy-induced neuropathy, radiation plexitis, surgical trauma) and paraneoplastic syndromes are less common causes
- Cancer patients are generally older and frailer than other chronic pain patients and may be more vulnerable to adverse drug effects
- First-line treatment with opioids is usual in this context but co-analgesics are almost certainly needed in addition.

9.1 Epidemiology

9.1.1 Limitations of existing studies

A recent systematic review on the epidemiology of cancer pain found that most studies of cancer pain prevalence do not categorize according to pathophysiology. That is, they do not specifically identify neuropathic pain. Recent developments in the definition and grading of neuropathic pain may improve future evidence, but categorization of pain remains a challenge. A review of pain in lung cancer (one of the commonest cancers to cause pain) similarly found that the causes or types of pain were infrequently described in the literature. Of 32 epidemiological pain studies identified, just four were classified by underlying cause of the pain and four by pathophysiological subtype.

9.1.2 Prevalence of cancer neuropathic pain

Despite these limitations, some conclusions can be drawn about the prevalence of cancer neuropathic pain. A prospective study of 2,266 cancer patients referred to a pain service identified neuropathic pain in 34%, with over two-thirds of these pains directly caused by the cancer, and one in seven related to cancer treatment. An international survey of cancer pain in 1,095 patients suggests that up to 40% of cancer pain may have a neuropathic component. This comprises 23% with a combination of somatic and neuropathic pain, 5% with a combination of somatic, visceral, and neuropathic pain, 4% combined visceral and neuropathic in origin, and only 8% purely neuropathic. Both of these studies may overestimate the prevalence of neuropathic pain because the study populations were selected groups: those referred to a pain service and consecutive patients identified by clinicians with an interest in cancer pain, respectively. Neuropathic pain is reported to occur in 25–32% of lung cancer patients, although again these figures may reflect a somewhat higher prevalence than in cancer patients overall, because of greater frequency of malignant invasion of neurological structures and of neurological damage from antineoplastic treatment in lung, as compared with other, cancers. Overall, one-third of cancer pains may have a neuropathic component, and mixed pathophysiology is much more frequent than 'pure' neuropathic pain.

9.1.3 Types of nerve damage

One detailed study of cancer neuropathic pain suggests that 79% of cases result from nerve compression, 16% from nerve injury, and 5% are sympathetically mediated. There is some indication that reversible nerve compression may eventually progress to irreversible nerve injury, and that nerve injury pain may itself be more difficult to treat than nerve compression pain. Sympathetically mediated pain is particularly challenging to manage, and may be better classed as a type of complex regional pain syndrome. The latter includes (but is not confined to) sympathetically mediated pain. Categorizing pain in this more detailed way is difficult, both in clinical and research contexts, and this evidence should therefore be interpreted with caution.

9.2 Clinical presentation

9.2.1 Direct tumour infiltration of peripheral nerves

This most commonly occurs with rib metastases, or with paravertebral or retroperitoneal metastases. Presentation is directly related to the exact nerve or nerves involved, and usually can be relatively easily related to known spread of the cancer, as long as suspicion of metastatic spread to the site concerned is high (see Box 9.1 for causes of cancer neuropathic pain).

9.2.2 Tumour infiltration of plexi

Cervical plexopathy is commonly due to head and neck tumours or cervical lymph node metastases. Pain may occur in the pre-auricular,

Box 9.1 Likely causes of cancer neuropathic pain

Predominantly acute pain

- Painful peripheral neuropathy due to chemotherapy toxicity (most commonly from vinca alkaloids, platinum compounds, or taxanes)
- Acute radiation-induced plexopathy or myelopathy.

Predominantly chronic pain

- *Direct tumour infiltration of a peripheral nerve*—most commonly from paravertebral or retroperitoneal spread, or from rib metastases
- *Tumour infiltration of a nerve plexus*—cervical plexopathy is most common in primary head and neck tumours or metastases to the neck, brachial plexopathy is most common in lymphoma, breast, or lung cancer, and lumbosacral plexopathy is most often seen with pelvic tumours
- *Radiculopathy*—due to tumour spread to involve dorsal spinal nerve roots, most often from epidural tumour mass or leptomeningeal metastases
- *Painful peripheral neuropathy*—may be due to direct tumour spread, chemotherapy toxicity, metabolic causes such as diabetes or renal or hepatic dysfunction, nutritional deficiencies, or paraneoplastic syndromes
- *Post-surgical pain syndromes*—post-mastectomy, post-thoracotomy, post-radical neck dissection, and phantom limb pain are the commonest examples
- *Post radiation pain syndromes*—these are uncommon and other causes of pain, such as recurrent tumour, should be considered first.

post-auricular, or anterior neck, and an associated ipsilateral Horner's syndrome or hemidiaphragmatic paralysis should be sought.

Brachial plexopathies occur usually as a result of axillary lymph node metastases in breast cancer or lymphoma, or because of direct extension of an apical lung cancer: Pancoast's tumour. They may present with upper plexus involvement (C5 and 6) or lower plexus involvement (C7, 8, and T1). In Pancoast's tumour, when there is direct extension from the lung apex, it is usually the lower plexus which is involved; pain often precedes neurological deficit and occurs particularly around the elbow, in the medial forearm, and fourth and fifth fingers.

Lumbosacral plexopathies are most often related to colorectal or cervical carcinomas, lymphomas, or metastases from breast cancer. Again, pain is often the first symptom, before any neurological deficit develops. Autonomic dysfunction is common, and motor and sensory deficits tend to occur subsequently. Pain presentation varies very much according to the part of the lumbosacral plexus involved, and may vary from pain in the back, low abdomen, flanks, and anterolateral thigh (upper plexus) to pain in the perineum, buttocks, and postero-lateral leg (lower plexus). Careful evaluation of lumbar and sacral neurological function is important, and deficits at multiple levels are usual.

9.2.3 **Radiculopathies**

Nerve damage to the dorsal spinal roots gives rise to radiculopathies. In cancer patients, this is most often caused by epidural tumour mass or leptomeningeal metastases. With epidural tumour mass, patients present with dermatomal pain in the affected territory; this tends to be unilateral in cervical and lumbosacral regions, and bilateral in the thorax. The pain is typically exacerbated by coughing or sneezing. Any presentation of this nature should lead to urgent consideration and investigation of associated spinal cord compression. Leptomeningeal metastases are less common, and may produce a variety of multifocal neurological symptoms and signs, including generalized headache and radicular pain in buttocks or lower back.

9.2.4 **Painful peripheral neuropathy**

The chemotherapeutic drugs associated with painful neuropathies are the vinca alkaloids (vinblastine, vincristine, vindesine, vinorelbine), platinum compounds (carboplatin, cisplatin, oxaliplatin), the taxanes (docetaxel and paclitaxel), procarbazine, and altretamine. Most of these agents, at usual doses, only infrequently cause painful neuropathies, but vincristine, vinorelbine, and cisplatin are more commonly problematic. Presentation is usually of painful or 'burning' hands or feet, with allodynia, hyperalgesia, or parasthesiae. A variety of sensory, motor, or autonomic deficits may be associated, and reduced tendon reflexes are common. Vinblastine and vincristine have also occasionally been linked to neuropathic jaw pain.

After discontinuation of the drug, symptoms usually subside slowly, although they may take several months to do so. Neuropathies associated with cisplatin may be more persistent. Thalidomide, although not a chemotherapeutic agent, is increasingly used in cancer patients, and may also cause painful peripheral neuropathy, usually reversible on stopping treatment.

9.2.5 **Paraneoplastic syndromes**

Paraneoplastic syndromes are themselves rare, occurring in just 6% of all cancer patients. Paraneoplastic sensory or sensorimotor neuropathies causing neuropathic pain are even less common, but are recognized most often in association with small-cell lung cancer, breast cancer, gynaecological malignancies, and myeloma. Patients usually present with an asymmetrical painful sensory or mixed sensorimotor neuropathy, but there is wide variation in both presentation and subsequent course. Metabolic or nutritional deficiencies may be a more likely cause of sensory neuropathies in cancer patients than paraneoplastic syndromes, and these should always be considered and excluded.

9.2.6 Post-surgical neuropathic pain

Neuropathic pain may also present following surgery; the commonest presentations are after mastectomy with axillary node dissection, post radical neck dissection, after thoracotomy, and phantom limb pain following amputation.

9.3 Assessment

9.3.1 Patient factors

A number of patient factors tend to make assessment and subsequent management of cancer neuropathic pain more challenging. These include:

- The generally older age of cancer patients
- The greater frailty and increased co-morbidity associated with older age
- The possible involvement of other organ systems in patients with advanced metastatic cancer (especially hepatic and renal impairment)
- The high frequency of cognitive impairment in patients with advanced cancer.

9.3.2 Identifying cancer neuropathic pain

As in non-cancer neuropathic pain, there is no single symptom or sign pathognomonic of cancer neuropathic pain. The infrequency of 'pure' neuropathic pain, and the fact that pain mechanisms are often mixed in cancer patients, means that it is particularly hard to achieve consistency in assessment. There is less agreement between independent assessors in the context of neuropathic pain compared to nociceptive pain, and it is often challenging to identify specific mechanisms and causes of pain in the individual patient. With cancer progression, different mechanisms may also change over time and the relationship between symptoms, signs, and mechanisms is unclear. It is best therefore to maintain a low threshold of suspicion for neuropathic pain, and actively seek out any features suggestive of neuropathic pain if:

- Any pain in a cancer patient is persistent or severe
- Any pain is particularly intense or distressing in quality
- Any pain does not respond to standard approaches
- The known anatomical location of disease suggests a neuropathic component or pain from nerve compression or injury is likely
- Treatment of the cancer has included one of the examples identified in Box 9.1.

Assessment tools may be helpful. In particular, the Leeds Assessment of Neuropathic Symptoms and Signs scale is simple and has been shown to be suitable for assessing neuropathic pain in cancer patients, although changes in skin appearance or colour may be less useful as an indicator of neuropathic pain in cancer patients.

9.3.3 **Other considerations**

In the history, it is important to identify co-morbidity, especially diabetes mellitus, and previous liver or renal disease, since these may increase the likelihood of painful peripheral neuropathy. A careful history of the cancer is also crucial, including results of any staging investigations, in order to clarify the known or suspected location of the primary tumour and any direct or secondary spread. Also important are the full details of any treatment received, including radiotherapy, chemotherapy (exact chemotherapeutic agents and doses used), and any surgical treatment. A detailed history of the pain, associated symptoms, and the impact on the patient and family is then required, with particular attention to the features identified in Table 9.1.

Table 9.1 Important features of assessment in cancer neuropathic pain	
Symptom or sign	Identify

Pain	• For both spontaneous and evoked pain:
	  • location and radiation
	  • pattern (onset, timing, and duration)
	  • quality
	  • severity or intensity
	  • triggers (for evoked pain).

Sensory symptoms	Abnormal sensations (crawling, prickling, itching, or tingling) Numbness
Sensory signs	Sensory loss Colour changes Allodynia (pain from normally non-noxious stimuli) Hyperalgesia (increased sensitivity to normally painful stimuli)
Motor symptoms and signs	Motor symptoms and signs are often present but can be subtle
Other considerations	**Explore**
Co-morbidity	Concurrent illness, and impact of metastatic disease on other systems
Prognosis	Expected course of disease— consider whether suspected cause of neuropathic pain is likely to worsen
Impact on quality of life	Overall function and disability Psychological and emotional effects Family impact

9.4 **Treatment**

9.4.1 **General approaches**

Management of cancer-related neuropathic pain is often challenging and a number of different therapeutic options may be required, either concurrently or sequentially. Pain brings its own psychological costs to the patient, but the additional psychological impact of prolonged titration and adjustment of medication, and changes in therapeutic approach, should not be underestimated. Clear and consistent explanation of proposed management to patient and family at each stage can make a major difference in lessening this impact and maintaining levels of trust between the patient and professionals.

In general, pharmacological management of cancer neuropathic pain draws heavily on evidence from studies in non-cancer conditions, and limited work has been done in patients with cancer neuropathic pain. However, there are some specific issues in cancer neuropathic pain which will be highlighted here.

9.4.2 **Opioids**

While there is good evidence that opioids are effective in non-cancer neuropathic pain, there is much less evidence in cancer neuropathic pain. What evidence there is suggests that the overall responsiveness of cancer neuropathic pain to opioids is less than for cancer nociceptive pain. However, the response of any individual patient cannot be predicted, and higher doses may be effective. A trial of opioid is therefore recommended first-line, but with the expectation that careful titration of doses upwards to effect or until intolerable side-effects intervene may be required. Co-analgesics are almost certainly needed alongside opioids (Box 9.2).

There is insufficient evidence to suggest that any one opioid has specific advantages over another. Given the absence of data, including lack of comparative studies and the wide individual variability in response to different opioids, a low threshold for switch to an alternative opioid is suggested. Combining two opioids may, in future, improve the management of cancer neuropathic pain, but research is needed to indicate which opioids or doses might be beneficial. Tramadol has noradrenergic and serotonergic activity, as well as opioid agonist activity—some have therefore suggested it may be of extra value in treatment of neuropathic pain, although there is little evidence to support or refute this suggestion.

9.4.3 **Antidepressants**

Limited evaluation of tricyclic antidepressants has taken place in cancer neuropathic pain. Most evidence is extrapolated from patients with diabetic neuropathy or postherpetic neuralgia. However, limited

Box 9.2 **Steps in the use of opioid analgesia in cancer neuropathic pain**

- Optimize the opioid regimen (no one opioid can be recommended above another)
- Titrate upwards until effect or intolerable side-effects.
- Maximally manage side-effects to allow for further titration if possible
- Ensure all appropriate non-pharmacological interventions have been considered
- If unacceptable opioid side-effects persist without adequate analgesic effect, consider:
  - adjuvant analgesics
  - switching to an alternative opioid.

existing evidence combined with extensive clinical experience suggests tricyclics are effective in this context, and there is also early indication that amitriptyline may have specific benefit for chemotherapy-related neuropathic symptoms. The main disadvantage of tricyclic antidepressants is frequent antimuscarinic side-effects, including cardiotoxicity, hypotension, and confusion, which are problematic in the elderly cancer patient or those with cardiac co-morbidity. Newer antidepressants such as venlafaxine may be better tolerated but show limited effectiveness.

9.4.4 **Antiepileptics**

There is considerable evidence to support the use of gabapentin and pregabalin in non-cancer neuropathic pain (although effectiveness is less clear in chemotherapy-induced neuropathic pain). Nevertheless, their effectiveness in non-cancer neuropathic pain has been extrapolated by clinicians to apply to cancer patients. One study has provided early evidence that gabapentin may be beneficial to patients with cancer neuropathic pain, but the side-effects of dizziness and sedation may limit dose titration because patients are frailer. Pregabalin side-effects may be greater still. In the light of possible synergistic effects between morphine and gabapentin, concurrent reduction of opioid doses may also be needed.

9.4.5 **Other pharmacological agents**

Several other agents have been suggested or used clinically for cancer neuropathic pain, but with little supporting evidence—the limited evidence almost all derives from other populations. There is some evidence, for instance, that ketamine is effective in post-traumatic neuropathic pain, and lidocaine 5% patches have been shown to have some benefit in peripheral neuropathic pain. Such agents are considered in more detail elsewhere in this book and may be considered for individual patients with severe and resistant cancer neuropathic pain. However, they should be used by specialist teams with experience in their use.

Key references

Bennett, M.I. (2005). Gabapentin significantly improves analgesia in people receiving opioids for neuropathic cancer pain. *Cancer Treat. Rev.*, **31** (1), 58–62. [Commentary on: Caraceni, A., Zecca, E., Bonezzi, C., Arcuri, E., Yaya Tur R., Maltoni, M. (2004). Gabapentin for neuropathic cancer pain: a randomized controlled trial for the Gabapentin Cancer Pain Study Group. *J. Clin. Oncol.*, **22**, 2909–17.]

Caraceni, A., and Portenoy, R.K. (1999). An international survey of cancer pain characteristics and syndromes. IASP Task Force on Cancer Pain. International Association for the Study of Pain. *Pain*, **82**(3), 263–74.

Cherny, N.I., Thaler, H.T., Friedlander-Klar, H., Lapin, J., Foley, K.M., Houde, R., *et al.* (1994). Opioid responsiveness of cancer pain syndromes caused by neuropathic or nociceptive mechanisms: a combined analysis of controlled, single-dose studies. *Neurology*, **44**(5), 857–61.

Goudas, L.C., Bloch, R., Gialeli-Goudas, M., Lau, J., and Carr D.B. (2005). The epidemiology of cancer pain. *Cancer Invest*, **23**(2), 182–90.

Grond, S., Zech, D., Diefenbach, C., Radbruch, L., and Lehmann, K.A. (1996). Assessment of cancer pain: a prospective evaluation in 2266 cancer patients referred to a pain service. *Pain*, **64**(1), 107–14.

Potter, J., and Higginson, I.J. (2004). Pain experienced by lung cancer patients: a review of prevalence, causes and pathophysiology. *Lung Cancer*, **43**(3), 247–57.

Potter, J., Higginson, I.J., Scadding, J.W., and Quigley, C. (2003). Identifying neuropathic pain in patients with head and neck cancer: use of the Leeds Assessment of Neuropathic Symptoms and Signs scale. *J. Roy. Soc. Med.*, **96**(8), 379–83.

Chapter 10

Neuropathic back pain

Rainer Freynhagen

> ### Key points
>
> - Approximately 25–30% of patients with chronic low back pain have a neuropathic component, most usually chronic lumbar radicular pain.
> - Distinguishing between radicular and pseudoradicular syndromes in low back pain may have some clinical relevance but in practice is difficult to achieve.
> - A neuropathic component in low back pain can be identified through a combination of verbal descriptors and thorough clinical examination including evoking nerve root tension signs or dural irritation (e.g. straight leg raise). There is poor correlation between radiologic imaging and clinical symptoms.
> - Treatment of chronic neuropathic low back pain is similar to other neuropathic pain conditions and should be tailored to the individual.

10.1 Background

Acute and chronic low back pain (LBP) is highly prevalent in the primary care setting and from large epidemiological studies it is known that between 20–35% of patients with back pain suffer from a neuropathic pain component. Chronic lumbar radicular pain is without doubt the most common neuropathic pain syndrome nowadays. The pathophysiology of back pain is complex and both nociceptive as well as neuropathic pain-generating mechanisms are thought to be involved, hence the term *mixed pain syndrome* is established in this context. Diagnosis and management of neuropathic LBP remains an enigma, mainly because of the lack of a gold standard for both. Accuracy of diagnostic tests used to identify the source of back pain and their usefulness in clinical practice, particularly for guiding treatment selection, is unclear. There are no standard treatment guidelines for neuropathic low back pain and treatment is still likely to be a trial-and-error process where comorbidities and concurrent medications should be considered. Moreover, back pain is one of the single most costly disorders in many industrialised nations, and neuropathic pain components add significantly to this cost.

10.2 Pathophysiology

10.2.1 Basic mechanisms

Nociceptive pain represents a normal biological mechanism for preventing, or limiting, tissue damage.

The nociceptive component results from activation of nociceptors that innervate ligaments, small joints, muscle and tendons. Neuropathic pain in contrast to nociceptive pain, is produced by damage to, or pathological changes in the peripheral or central nervous system. Simultaneous neuropathic involvement in low-back pain may be caused by lesions of nociceptive sprouts within the degenerated disc (local neuropathic pain), mechanical compression of the nerve root (mechanical neuropathic root pain), or by action of inflammatory mediators such as chemokines and other cytokines (inflammatory neuropathic root pain), which can originate from the degenerative disc even without any mechanical compression. Hence, a variety of nerve-damaging stimuli are likely to generate a neuropathic pain component in patients presenting with chronic back pain.

10.2.2 Radiculopathy and pseudoradiculopathy

Radicular and pseudoradicular syndromes were often considered to be distinct entities. The rationale behind this distinction stems from the hypothesis that pain from local proximal disorders that do not affect any nerves or nerve roots, i.e. facet joint disease, piriformis syndrome, might be perceived in proximal dermatomes within the thigh (referred pain) whereas pain from disorders associated with nerve root compression is often felt in distal dermatomes below the knee (projected pain). The distinction of both clinical features is thought to be clinically and therapy-relevant, however, given the present level of understanding, it is not possible to differentiate clearly between both in a large number of patients.

Radicular pain is defined as a pain that radiates below the knee along the dermatome of a nerve (sensory distribution) due to inflammation or other irritation of the nerve root at its connection to the spinal column (see Figure 10.1 left). A common form is sciatica for which the first cited use of the word was registered in 1450. Nerve root compression by a protruded intervertebral disk or an inflammatory

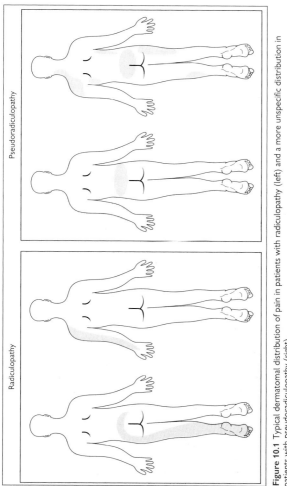

Figure 10.1 Typical dermatomal distribution of pain in patients with radiculopathy (left) and a more unspecific distribution in patients with pseudoradiculopathy (right).

Radiculopathy

Pseudoradiculopathy

etiology (e.g. leakage of inflammatory mediators from a ruptured nucleus pulposus) are suspected to be the main causes of sciatic pain. However, sciatica is more a set of symptoms rather than a diagnosis for what is irritating the root of the nerve, and causes are manyfold (see Table 10.1). Even the sympathetic nervous system is considered to be involved in causing radicular pain in man while neuroanatomical and immunohistochemical studies revealed sympathetic neurones in the intervertebral disc and adjacent tissue. It is important to keep in mind that symptoms will often be different depending upon the underlying cause.

Pseudoradicular pain is defined as pain that mimics true nerve root irritation. It also extends to the legs or arms but never reaches the foot or fingers and it cannot be allocated to any nerve root (see Figure 10.1 right). It is usually attributed to non-nerve related structures and mechanical factors, musculoskeletal dysfunctions, degenerative changes in connective tissues and local or even systemic inflammation are commonly regarded as the main reasons for pseudoradicular syndromes. Pseudoradicular pain might be perceived in proximal dermatomes and is then called 'referred pain'.

10.3 **Epidemiology and costs of neuropathic back-pain**

From current large epidemiological studies, between 20–35% of patients with back pain suffer from a neuropathic pain component. They are substantially more frequent in persons with more severe

Table 10.1 Causes of radiculopathy and pseudoradiculopathy (in the order of estimated prevalence)	
Radiculopathy	**Pseudoradiculopathy**
Herniated disc with nerve compression	Sprained muscular conditions
Lumbar spinal stenosis (elderly adults)	Facet joint syndromes
Foraminal stenosis (elderly adults)	Diseases of the sacroiliac joint (ISG-joint)
Diabetes mellitus	Blockages of the lumbar spinal column
Degenerative disc disease	Osteochondrosis
Scar tissue from previous spinal surgery	Inflammation of the trochanteric bursa (Bursitis)
Nerve root injuries	Local or systemic inflammation
Spondylolisthesis	Stroke (can mimic a sacral radiculopathy)

grades of back pain compared with persons with mild back pain. Analysis of claims recorded in a US health-insurance database indicated that back and neck pain with neuropathic involvement is probably the most frequent neuropathic disorder.

New research data from Germany which modelled the relative prevalence and cost of neuropathic pain in back-pain patients in the general population suggest that almost one in five persons with back pain experience symptoms indicative of a neuropathic pain component. Given that the proportion of all persons in the general population with back pain is about one-third, the number with neuropathic back pain components corresponds to about 6% of the general population, which means almost 6 million patients only in Germany. This estimate is consistent with data from UK and French studies (see Chapter 3). Moreover, it has been shown, that neuropathic pain components are a significant cost factor in back pain. On average, the typical costs associated with a person suffering neuropathic back pain are approximately 50% higher than those of an average patient, and even 70% higher than the cost of a patient with non-neuropathic back pain. On the basis of the German data it has been estimated that the total costs of back pain to the German society add up to €48.9 bn and the total (direct plus indirect) costs incurred only by the subpopulation with neuropathic aetiology aggregates to €13 bn.

10.4 **Screening and diagnostic approaches**

In the diagnostic work-up of back pain a thorough neurological examination is absolutely essential. In addition to clinical bedside examination that specifically try to evoke nerve root tension signs or dural irritation (e.g. tendon reflexes, sensibility and motor function, active flexion in standing position with a passive cervical flexion, a straight-leg raising test with a passive dorsiflexion of the foot, straight-leg raising test with a passive cervical flexion), radiological exams and neurophysiological tesing is often used to determine a nerve lesion or nerve compression in these patients to document the radicular component. These approaches might, however, be inconclusive as previous studies have shown poor correlation between radiologic imaging and clinical symptoms and even neurophysiologic tests lack specificity.

Many clinicians that manage patients with chronic back pain do not have adequate skill or even the time for such a diagnostic approach, especially in primary care. Neither do they have easy access to electrophysiology or Quantitative sensory testing (QST) and so it makes sense to exploit the value of verbal descriptors and pain qualities as a basis for distinguishing neuropathic pain from other types of chronic pain.

Patients typically present with specific symptoms expressed with a certain intensity rather than easily recognizable neurological lesions. Therefore in the last 5 years, much research has been undertaken to develop easy to handle screening tools for this purpose which are based on verbal pain description with, or without, limited bedside testing (see Chapter 5). In particular, one such tool (pain*DETECT* Figure 10.2) was developed in a population of patients with low back pain and has shown good discriminant validity.

In a recent study using Quantitative Sensory Testing (QST, see Chapter 4), which is a reliable psychophysical test of large- and small-fiber sensory modalities referring to a set of methods that extend the traditional neurological examination of somatosensory function, it was demonstrated that even pseudoradicular back pain can be associated with subclinical sensory deficits in the distal extremity. Obviously many back pain patients suffer from a clinically unrecognized neuropathic pain component which may result in a suboptimal treatment since neuropathic pain requires a different therapeutic first-line approach.

10.5 Treatment of neuropathic back pain

Since the rationale for separating neuropathic pain from non-neuropathic pain has direct implications for treatment, it is of the utmost importance for the clinician to identify the severity of the different pain components in each individual patient. Researchers and clinicians are trying hard to develop early, intensive treatments that target the molecular and cellular mechanisms involved in neuropathic pain or, ideally, prevent it from occurring in the first place. This 'mechanism-based approach' may become reality in the future but physicians are currently faced with a myriad of options when choosing treatment for neuropathic back pain, none of which have been shown to be effective for all patients. Little consensus exists on primary treatment choices and in the interim, evidence-based guidelines for the pharmacological management of neuropathic pain must provide guidance for selecting first-, second- and third-line medications that offer acceptable control alone or in combination, and allow clinicians to bridge the gap between current knowledge and clinical application.

Two guidelines have recently been published by the Canadian Pain Society and the European Federation of Neurological Societies, which have evaluated the existing evidence on the pharmacological treatment of NeP using a comprehensive review of the literature. Both guidelines attempt to guide physicians in choosing evidence-based treatments supported by well designed clinical trials. However, both guidelines emphasise that a modern treatment choice must include individual patient factors as adverse effects, comorbidities such as poor sleep, depressed mood, and anxiety and quality of life, as well as the effects on pain, symptoms and signs. Undeniably, the goal of NeP management is not only to alleviate pain but also to treat the patient as a whole. The available evidence suggests that in these cases antidepressants and/or anticonvulsants in combination with either opioids, traditional non-steroidal anti-inflammatory drugs or muscle relaxants could be useful.

Key references

Attal N., Cruccu G., Haanpaa M., Hansson P., Jensen T.S., Nurmikko T., Sampaio C., Sindrup S., Wiffen P. (2006) EFNS guidelines on pharmacological treatment of neuropathic pain. *Eur J Neurol*, **13**(11), 1153–69.

Baron R., Binder A. (2004) How neuropathic is sciatica? The mixed pain concept. *Orthopade*, **33**(5), 568–75.

Bennett M.I., Attal N., Backonja M.M., Baron R., Bouhassira D., Freynhagen R., Scholz J., Tolle T.R., Wittchen H.U., Jensen T.S. (2007) Using screening tools to identify neuropathic pain. *Pain*, **127**(3), 199–203.

Bennett M.I., Bouhassira D. (2007) Epidemiology of neuropathic pain: can we use the screening tools? *Pain*, 132(1–2), 12–13.

Freynhagen R., Baron R., Gockel U., Tolle T.R. (2006) painDETECT: a new screening questionnaire to identify neuropathic components in patients with back pain. *Curr Med Res Opin*, **22**(10), 1911–20.

Freynhagen R., Rolke R., Baron R., Tolle T.R., Rutjes A.K., Schu S., Treede R.D. (2008) Pseudoradicular and radicular low-back pain — a disease continuum rather than different entities? Answers from quantitative sensory testing. *Pain*, **135**(1–2), 65–74.

Freynhagen R., and Baron R. (2009) The evaluation of neuropathic components in low back pain. *Curr Pain Headache Rep.* Jun; **13**(3), 185–90

Freynhagen R., and Bennett M.I. (2009) Diagnosis and management of neuropathic pain. *BMJ*. 338:b3002 [in press].

Moulin D.E., Clark A.J., Gilron I., Ware M.A., Watson C.P., Sessle B.J., Coderre T., Morley-Forster P.K., Stinson J., Boulanger A., Peng P., Finley G.A., Taenzer P., Squire P., Dion D., Cholkan A., Gilani A., Gordon A., Henry J., Jovey R., Lynch M., Mailis-Gagnon A., Panju A., Rollman G.B., Velly A. (2007) Pharmacological management of chronic neuropathic pain—Consensus statement and guidelines from the Canadian Pain Society. *Pain Res Manag*, **12**(1), 13–21.

Schmidt C.O., Schweikert B., Wenig C.M., Schmidt U., Gockel U., Freynhagen R., Tölle T.R., Baron R., Kohlmann T. (2009) *Eur J Pain*. Feb 5 [Epub ahead of print].

painDETECT™ **PAIN QUESTIONNAIRE**

Date: _ _ _ _ _ _ _ _ Patient: Last name: _ _ _ _ _ _ _ First name: _ _ _ _ _ _ _

How would you assess your pain   now , at this moment?

0 1 2 3 4 5 6 7 8 9 10
none   max.

How strong was the   strongest   pain during the past 4 weeks?

0 1 2 3 4 5 6 7 8 9 10
none   max.

How strong was the pain during the past 4 weeks   on average ?

0 1 2 3 4 5 6 7 8 9 10
none   max.

Please mark your
main area of pain

Mark the picture that best describes
the course of your pain:

Persistent pain with
slight fluctuations ☐

Persistent pain with pain
attacks ☐

Pain attacks without
pain between them ☐

Pain attacks with pain
between them ☐

Does your pain radiate to other regions of your
body?   yes ☐   no ☐
If yes, please draw the direction in
which the pain radiates.

Do you suffer from a burning sensation (e.g., stinging nettles) in the marked areas?
never ☐   hardly noticed ☐   slightly ☐   moderately ☐   strongly ☐   very strongly ☐

Do you have a tingling or prickling sensation in the area of your pain (like crawling ants or electrical tingling)?
never ☐   hardly noticed ☐   slightly ☐   moderately ☐   strongly ☐   very strongly ☐

Is light touching (clothing, a blanket) in this area painful?
never ☐   hardly noticed ☐   slightly ☐   moderately ☐   strongly ☐   very strongly ☐

Do you have sudden pain attacks in the area of your pain, like electric shocks?
never ☐   hardly noticed ☐   slightly ☐   moderately ☐   strongly ☐   very strongly ☐

Is cold or heat (bath water) in this area occasionally painful?
never ☐   hardly noticed ☐   slightly ☐   moderately ☐   strongly ☐   very strongly ☐

Do you suffer from a sensation of numbness in the areas that you marked?
never ☐   hardly noticed ☐   slightly ☐   moderately ☐   strongly ☐   very strongly ☐

Does slight pressure in this area, e.g., with a finger, trigger pain?
never ☐   hardly noticed ☐   slightly ☐   moderately ☐   strongly ☐   very strongly ☐

(To be filled out by the physician)

never	hardly noticed	slightly	moderately	strongly	very strongly
x 0 =	x 1 =	x 2 =	x 3 =	x 4 =	x 5 =

Total score ☐☐ out of 35

Figure 10.2 The pain*DETECT* screening tool incorporates a reliable and easy to use patient-based self-report questionnaire with 9 items that do not require a clinical examination (left page) and a quick scoring page for the physician.

painDETECT SCORING OF PAIN QUESTIONNAIRE

Date: Patient: Last name: First name:

Please transfer the total score from the pain questionnaire:

Total score

Please add up the following numbers, depending on the marked pain behavior pattern and the pain radiation. Then total up the final score:

	Persistent pain with slight fluctuations	0	
	Persistent pain with pain attacks	−1	if marked, or
	Pain attacks without pain between them	+1	if marked, or
	Pain attacks with pain between them	+1	if marked
	Radiating pain?	+2	if yes

Final score

Screening Result

Final score

| negative | unclear | positive |

0 1 2 3 4 5 6 7 8 9 10 11 12 13 14 15 16 17 18 19 20 21 22 23 24 25 26 27 28 29 30 31 32 33 34 35 36 37 38

A neuropathic pain component is unlikely (< 15%)

Result is ambiguous, however a neuropathic pain component can be present

A neuropathic pain component is likely (> 90%)

Figure 10.2 (Contd.)

Chapter 11

Antidepressants and antiepileptics for neuropathic pain

Henry J. McQuay and Philip Wiffen

Key points

- Antidepressants and antiepileptics are well-established treatments for neuropathic pain
- Clinical trial evidence can be limited in both scope of neuropathic pain conditions studied and duration of treatment. This leaves prescribers to extrapolate evidence to other conditions, and without information on longer-term effects
- Lack of head-to-head comparisons results in the use of indirect evidence such as NNTs, but the sample size used to derive NNT values is equally important
- Although tricyclics appear more effective than other classes of antidepressants, this needs to be balanced against higher incidence of adverse effects
- League tables suggest that the character of the neuropathic pain, whether it be burning or shooting, does not determine its responsiveness to either of the drug classes.

11.1 Introduction

11.1.1 Background to antidepressants and antiepileptics

The first reports of antiepileptic efficacy in trigeminal neuralgia go back nearly 50 years, and tricyclic antidepressant efficacy was also shown in a variety of pain syndromes decades ago. Our concern now is not whether antidepressants and antiepileptics work in neuropathic pain, although we still have to show that for any new drugs that come along, but how well do the different drugs within the antidepressant and antiepileptic categories work compared with each other, and indeed how well do antidepressants work compared with antiepileptics? The other side of the coin is the relative adverse effect burden within and between the two drug classes. Exactly how effective the two drug classes are, and at what cost in adverse effects, remains a focus of attention for clinicians, researchers, and the patients themselves.

11.1.2 Antidepressant pharmacology

Tricyclic antidepressants (TCAs) such as amitriptyline and imipramine have a multimodal mechanism of action. They inhibit pre-synaptic uptake of serotonin and noradrenaline, interact with sodium and calcium ion channels, and block some post-synaptic histamine and muscarinic receptors. Tricyclics generally show non-linear pharmacokinetics, meaning that there is no linear relationship between drug dose and steady state serum concentration. For example, a 30-fold difference in serum concentrations has been observed on the same TCA dose in different patients. This can also result in significantly higher serum concentrations (and clinical effects) despite small dose changes, and vice versa. Dry mouth, drowsiness, and postural hypotension are the most frequent adverse effects and are often more pronounced in the elderly. In general, sub-antidepressant doses of TCAs can produce analgesic benefit; the usual starting dose of amitriptyline is 25mg daily, titrated to a mean of around 75mg.

More selective antidepressants include selective serotonin re-uptake inhibitors (SSRIs) such as paroxetine and fluoxetine, and balanced serotonin noradrenaline re-uptake inhibitors (SNRIs) such as venlafaxine and the more potent duloxetine (the latter is licensed for painful diabetic neuropathy). Both these drug classes have virtually no blocking effects on post-synaptic receptors or ion channels, leading to fewer side-effects. A current debate is to what extent the multimodal action of TCAs contributes to their apparent superiority, as well as greater adverse effects, compared with SSRIs and SNRIs in treating neuropathic pain.

11.1.3 Antiepileptic pharmacology

The mechanism of action of older antiepileptic drugs, such as phenytoin and carbamazepine, was thought to occur via blockade of voltage-dependent sodium channels. However, recent work suggests that carbamazepine may in fact have additional actions via serotonergic pathways (which is not surprising as it is structurally very similar to TCAs). Newer antiepileptics, such as gapapentin, pregabalin, and lamotrigine, have actions on various receptors, including the $\alpha_2\delta$ subunit of voltage-dependent calcium channels and modulation of GABA synthesis, release, and metabolism. Adverse effects are similar for all antiepileptics and those most frequently reported are drowsiness, fatigue, and ataxia. Longer-term adverse effects are not always apparent in clinical trials of short duration, and weight gain associated with gabapentin is an example of this. Doses of antiepileptics used to treat neuropathic pain are generally similar to those used in epilepsy. (See also Chapter 12 for parenteral use of antiepileptic drugs.)

11.2 Clinical trial evidence

11.2.1 Issues of scope

The focus on the relative efficacy and adverse effect rates of the two drug classes has made us think more about neuropathic pain in general, and about the trials, their conduct, and outcomes used in reporting them. A simple example of the wider issues is whether or not you include fibromyalgia as a neuropathic pain symptom. It responds to the same drug classes but is unlike other neuropathic pain syndromes in that there is no demonstrable nervous system dysfunction.

Most of the trials from which the information below was drawn were done in post-herpetic neuralgia (PHN) and painful diabetic neuropathy (PDN). These two conditions are relatively easy to diagnose and have therefore become the test-bed of choice for testing drug efficacy in neuropathic pain. But most neuropathic pain is not PHN or PDN. Historically, drug remedies for PHN and PDN have been effective in other neuropathic pain syndromes, but we do not know if negative results in PHN and PDN are predictive of lack of efficacy in other neuropathic pain syndromes. Much of our prescribing for neuropathic pain involves this kind of extrapolation from results in other, different, pain syndromes.

11.2.2 Issues of duration

For the trials themselves one of the major questions is how long— weeks or months—should the drug be studied for us to be certain of its efficacy. Many neuropathic pain syndromes may need medication for years, so that issues of efficacy and safety over the longer term are important to patients and prescribers. Most of the trials, however, are of less than 8 weeks' duration, and it is only for the very recently introduced drugs that we have information for up to 3 months of treatment. Even this is limited in relation to the duration of the condition. We just do not know the proportion of patients in whom initial drug efficacy subsequently wanes and over what period any such waning occurs. Neither do we know the corollary, the proportion in whom initial drug efficacy is maintained without dose escalation for one or indeed 5 years.

Technically, neuropathic pain trials may be difficult trials to run because for many of the antidepressant and antiepileptic drugs there has to be a titration to the optimal dose for maximal effect and minimal adverse effects, and trial designs necessarily become complicated to incorporate this titration. The alternative (using fixed doses of these drugs) risks underdosing some patients and overdosing others, as well as underestimating efficacy and overestimating adverse effects.

11.3 **Determining relative efficacy**

11.3.1 **Lack of head-to-head (direct) evidence**

There are surprisingly few head-to-head comparisons of antidepressants and antiepileptics in neuropathic pain, and even fewer head-to-head comparisons either between different antidepressants or between different antiepileptics. Indeed, the small numbers of patients studied in these conditions may come as a surprise. An example is that all the sweeping statements made about the lack of efficacy of SSRIs in neuropathic pain are based on the grand total of 80 patients studied in trials of good quality, and in one of those trials the SSRI did just as well as the tricyclic antidepressant. Perhaps the emergence of medical myths is in inverse proportion to the amount of data.

In the only modern head-to-head comparison, a small study of 19 patients who crossed over between gabapentin (up to 1800mg) and amitriptyline (up to 75mg) in painful diabetic neuropathy found that there was no significant difference in pain scores with the two drugs, or in global ratings of pain relief (52% with at least moderate pain relief during gabapentin and 67% during amitriptyline) ($P > 0.1$). Both treatments caused similar rates of adverse events.

11.3.2 **Using systematic review (indirect) evidence**

In the absence of head-to-head or direct comparisons of these drugs in neuropathic pain, how are we to arrive at an assessment of the relative efficacy and tolerability of the different drugs? Earlier reviews and the most recent updates have used systematic review techniques to gather the data from good-quality trials comparing antiepileptics or antidepressants with placebo, the indirect method. The efficacy of the different drugs against placebo is then calculated and expressed as the number-needed-to-treat (NNT). The NNT values of the different drugs may then be compared to determine the relative efficacy of the different drugs.

An analogy might be that we want to know who is the quickest runner in the room. We could simply make everyone run 100 metres, competing with each other in one race, the direct method. This would be the head-to-head comparison. We could alternatively get each individual to run 100 metres against the clock and on their own. We could then compare the times to work out who was quickest. This latter indirect method is the equivalent of deriving the relative efficacy by comparing each drug's performance against placebo. To estimate the relative efficacy of antiepileptics and antidepressants in neuropathic pain, we do not have a choice. We do not have direct comparisons, so we have to use an indirect method.

11.3.3 Limitations of indirect methods

These direct and indirect methods of assessing the efficacy of drugs used to manage neuropathic pain produce remarkably similar estimates, so one need not apologize for using the indirect technique. It is important, however, to be aware of the weaknesses, and of these by far the most significant is size. If the performance of the drug or even the drug class is based on a small number of patients studied, then the estimate of that performance should be treated with caution. An estimate of efficacy derived from 500 patients compared with placebo is likely to be a great deal more robust than one obtained on just 80 patients.

This sounds obvious and is obvious, but it is forgotten constantly, and casual mention of the NNT value for a particular treatment in neuropathic pain without reference to the size of the sample from which it was derived is misleading at the very least (see Chapter 18 for further discussion of NNT values). Figure 11.1 (taken from Finnerup *et al.*, 2005) shows the range of NNT values in peripheral neuropathic pain for a number of antidepressant and antiepileptic drugs. The diameter of the point estimate for each drug is proportional to the number of patients on whom the estimate is based, and the number is printed beside the estimate.

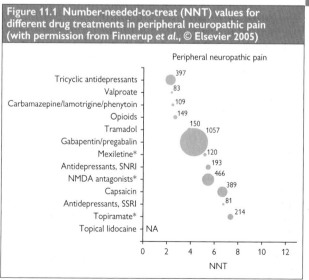

Figure 11.1 Number-needed-to-treat (NNT) values for different drug treatments in peripheral neuropathic pain (with permission from Finnerup *et al.*, © Elsevier 2005)

11.3.4 **Comparing different antidepressant classes**

For tricyclic antidepressants, an NNT estimate of just over 2 means that roughly one patient in two treated with a tricyclic antidepressant for their peripheral neuropathic pain will achieve at least 50% pain relief. The other patient might have some relief, but not enough to take them past the 50% relief mark. The estimate is based on roughly 400 patients. These patients may have been on different antidepressants, and at different doses. The different doses should not be too much of a problem because the dose for each patient should have been the optimal dose. If we are hypercritical and insist on splitting the efficacy estimate into the individual tricyclic drugs, then we will have little data for most of the individual drugs.

The NNT estimate with SSRI antidepressants is over 6, meaning that just one patient in 6 treated with an SSRI antidepressant for their peripheral neuropathic pain will achieve at least 50% pain relief, much worse than for the TCAs. Again the other 5 patients on the SSRI might have had some relief, but did not achieve 50% relief. The estimate is based on just 81 patients, and is in stark contrast to the more than 1,000 patients studied on gabapentin with an NNT estimate of just over 4. The smaller the point estimate in the figure, the less robust the estimate.

11.3.5 **The need for more clinical trials**

It has to be a concern that we have so little data on which to base important prescribing decisions. Using the antidepressants as an example, we would argue that SSRIs have not been adequately tested in neuropathic pain. The potential advantage of the lower adverse effect incidence with these drugs means perhaps that we need trials of adequate size and quality to check whether it really is true to say that SSRIs do not work in neuropathic pain. The number needed to harm (NNH) for trial withdrawal due to adverse effects of TCAs compared with placebo was estimated by Finnerup et al. at 14.7 (10.2–25.2). In contrast there was no statistically significant difference between SSRI and placebo for withdrawal due to adverse effects.

Interestingly, the efficacy NNT values for the mixed SNRIs, tested in modern trials of high quality, are, at around 4, very similar to the NNTs for gabapentin, and, like SSRIs, the adverse effect profile of the SNRIs is better than TCAs, with no statistically significant difference for withdrawal due to adverse effects compared with placebo. It is also possible that the 'best buy' status of TCAs in the relative efficacy league table may be due to overestimation of benefit in older small trials, some of crossover design.

Against that interpretation, however, is the finding that in both painful polyneuropathy and post-herpetic neuralgia there is a trend towards better effect of balanced serotonin and noradrenaline re-uptake inhibitors than of the mainly noradrenergic drugs. It will take fresh trials rather than meta-analysis to resolve the truth of the teaching of the past decades that the pharmacological 'shotgun' or multiple receptor action of the TCAs is more effective in neuropathic pain than the more selective or 'rifle' drugs.

11.4 Using relative efficacy

11.4.1 League tables

Diagnosing neuropathic pain is not difficult until people make it complicated. The combination of pain in an area of altered nervous system function, sometimes associated with pain on non-painful stimulus or excessive pain with a not very painful stimulus, and with a muted response to conventional analgesics, leads most clinicians to think of initiating treatment with antidepressant or antiepileptic. The choices of which drug class to use for initial treatment, and which particular drug to use within that drug class, are where the league table of relative efficacy can help. The term 'league table' is used to mean a ranking of the NNT efficacy values of the different drugs, where the lowest value is best and the highest worst (Figure 11.1).

We can now add data for at least 50% pain relief with duloxetine or pregabalin (Table 11.1). Pregabalin 600 mg is clearly more effective than 150 or 300 mg, with NNT values for 50% pain relief in postherpetic neuralgia (PHN) and painful diabetic neuropathy (DN) between 3 and 4. The dose-response with duloxetine in painful diabetic neuropathy is less clear.

The league table is of course based on results from many patients, whereas you are treating an individual patient, and takes little or no account of the adverse effects which are so important for chronic

Table 11.1 NNT data for duloxetine and pregabalin			
	Participants	NNT	95%CI
Duloxetine 60mg DN	1211	5.8	4.5 to 8.4
Duloxetine 120mg DN	1410	5.7	4.5 to 5.7
Pregabalin 150mg PHN	342	5.7	3.9 to 10
Pregabalin 300mg PHN	348	5.4	3.8 to 9.5
Pregabalin 300mg DN	529	6.1	(4.1 to 12)
Pregabalin 600mg PHN	356	3.3	(2.4 to 4.6)
Pregabalin 600mg DN	955	3.9	(3.2 to 5)

therapy. Nonetheless we have to start somewhere, and the league table provides us with the probability of success and the extent of that success for the different drugs so that we can make more informed decisions.

11.4.2 Treatment algorithm for antidepressants and antiepileptics

The algorithm produced by Finnerup *et al.* (Figure 11.2) is a practical example of where this process of meta-analysis can take us in the management of neuropathic pain. The algorithm attempts to encapsulate the evidence into a decision tree. The reality is that we lack the 'head-to-head' drug comparison studies necessary to put more flesh on the bones of the algorithm, and we lack understanding

Figure 11.2 Algorithm for sequence of different drug treatments in peripheral neuropathic pain (with permission from Finnerup et al. © Elsevier 2005)

as to whether different mechanisms underlying various neuropathic pain syndromes mean that we should have a different algorithm for each condition. For instance, standard teaching used to be that one would use an antidepressant for a burning pain and an antiepileptic for a shooting pain. There is little evidence to support this adage and indeed some evidence which goes against it, suggesting that the character of the pain, whether it be burning or shooting, does not determine its responsiveness to either of the drug classes.

A thought-provoking paper from Denmark suggests that current methods of dividing neuropathic pain and thinking of different underlying mechanisms does not help in predicting response to the different drugs. Intriguingly, the patients who did not respond to imipramine (the test TCA) tended not to respond well to the second-line drug, the antiepileptic gabapentin. For the moment it is one algorithm for all the different mechanisms underlying peripheral neuropathic pain.

Key references

Finnerup, N.B., Otto, M., McQuay, H.J., Jensen, T.S., and Sindrup, S.H. (2005). Algorithm for neuropathic pain treatment: an evidence-based proposal. *Pain*, **118**, 289–305.

Morello, C.M., Leckband, S.G., and Stoner, C.P. (1999). Randomized double-blind study comparing the efficacy of gabapentin with amitriptyline on diabetic peripheral neuropathy pain. *Arch Intern Med*, **159**, 1931–7.

Rasmussen, P.V., Sindrup, S.H., Jensen, T.S., and Bach, F.W. (2004). Therapeutic outcome in neuropathic pain: relationship to evidence of nervous system lesion. *Eur J Neurol*, **11**, 545–53.

Saarto, T. and Wiffen, P.J. (2005). Antidepressants for neuropathic pain. Cochrane Database of Systematic Reviews; CD005454.

Sindrup, S.H., Otto, M., Finnerup, N.B., and Jensen, T.S. (2005). Antidepressants in the treatment of neuropathic pain. *Basic Clin Pharmacol Toxicol*, **96**, 399–409.

Sultan A, Gaskell H, Derry S, Moore RA (2008). Duloxetine for painful diabetic neuropathy and fibromyalgia pain: systematic review of randomised trials. *BMC Neurol*, **8**(1), 29.

Wiffen, P., Collins, S., McQuay, H., Carroll, D., Jadad, A., and Moore, A. (2005). Anticonvulsant drugs for acute and chronic pain. Cochrane Database of Systematic Reviews; CD001133.

Wiffen, P.J., McQuay, H.J., Edwards, J.E., and Moore, R.A. (2005). Gabapentin for acute and chronic pain. Cochrane Database of Systematic Reviews; CD005452.

Wiffen, P.J., McQuay, H.J., and Moore, R.A. (2005). Carbamazepine for acute and chronic pain. Cochrane Database of Systematic Reviews; CD005451.

Wiffen P, Straube S, Derry S, Moore A, McQuay HJ (2008). Pregabalin for acute and chronic pain. Cochrane Database of Systematic Reviews (in press).

Chapter 12

Local anaesthetics and other pharmacological approaches

Gary McCleane

Key points

- While antidepressants, antiepileptics, and opioids form the mainstay of neuropathic pain management, alternative approaches are needed because not all patients respond to these drugs and side-effects can limit their use in others
- Topically applied drugs such a lidocaine 5% patches and capsaicin cream can produce local analgesic effects, though lidocaine is better tolerated
- Baclofen and tizanidine are conventionally used as skeletal muscle relaxants but can be effective neuropathic pain agents
- The analgesic effects of cannabinoids have not been as significant as were initially expected
- Intravenous fosphenytoin and lidocaine are useful adjuncts for reducing acute flare-ups of neuropathic pain.

While the conventional pharmacological treatment of neuropathic pain revolves around the use of the opioid analgesics, tricyclic anti-depressants, and antiepileptic drugs, a variety of other pharmacological entities outside these groups are used successfully in some patients with neuropathic pain.

12.1 Topical agents

12.1.1 Role of topical agents

Many patients like the concept of applying medication to the site where discomfort is felt. Of course, in the case of neuropathic pain this may not actually be where the abnormal neural function that generates the pain is occurring. Nevertheless, there are some neuropathic pain conditions where the abnormal process is either peripherally located from the start, or where peripheral neural changes occur as a result of a more central neural dysfunction. In these cases, peripheral application of a variety of agents can produce pain relief.

When drugs are applied topically, the effect can be due to either a localized peripheral effect, to a more central effect consequent on systemic absorption of the drug, or a combination of both. This chapter concentrates on drugs with a predominantly peripheral effect. Examples of those with a transdermal application but with predominantly central effects, such as transdermal fentanyl and buprenorphine, are covered elsewhere (see Chapter 14).

12.1.2 **Lidocaine**

The numbing effect of local anaesthetics occurs because of the sodium channel-blocking effect of the local anaesthetic in question. This numbing effect is easily achieved by infiltration of the local anaesthetic into the skin. However, such use of a local anaesthetic is impractical in those suffering from neuropathic pain. Fortunately, a simple method of topical local anaesthetic deposition exists in the form of the lidocaine 5% patch. This is applied to the area over which the pain is experienced, with only a small proportion of lidocaine that is contained in the patch being absorbed through the skin. That which is absorbed is enough in some cases to provide pain relief. Because of the small amounts of lidocaine actually absorbed, systemic side-effects do not occur.

Lidocaine 5% patch has been well verified in the treatment of post-herpetic neuralgia, but can also be a useful treatment in a wide variety of neuropathic and other pain conditions. Time to effect is measured in hours to a few days.

An added advantage of the lidocaine 5% patch is that it forms a physical barrier between the skin and, for example, clothing, which can reduce the discomfort of clothing rubbing against an area where allodynia, a common symptom of neuropathic pain, is experienced.

12.1.3 **Capsaicin**

Capsaicin, derived from the chilli pepper, has been used in medicinal practice for over 150 years. Repeated application results in absorption of capsaicin into peripheral nerves and axonal transport to the synaptic endings within the dorsal horn. Pain reduction is achieved by the propensity of capsaicin to inhibit the release of substance P from nerve endings and to reduce the density of epidermal nerve fibres. Because these effects are gradual and reversible, the time to effect can be at least 2 weeks and on occasions up to 4 weeks, and can occur only with repetitive and consistent application. Clearly it is only

> **Box 12.1 Strategies to minimize side-effects with capsaicin**
>
> - Apply in small volumes only
> - Use disposable gloves for application
> - Persist with application, if possible, as discomfort of application usually diminishes with time
> - Surround areas of application with petroleum jelly to prevent application outside the reference area
> - Pre-treatment with a topical local anaesthetic (e.g. EMLA®, or tetracaine (amethocaine) gel) can minimize application discomfort
> - Addition of gylceryl trinitrate ointment to capsaicin cream reduces application discomfort and can enhance the analgesic effect of the capsaicin.

of potential value where the pain is of peripheral origin and covers a relatively small area. Capsaicin cream is commercially available in 0.025% and 0.075% concentrations.

The most common adverse effect associated with capsaicin application is a burning, tingling discomfort at the site of application along with mechanical and thermal allodynia. Usually these unpleasant effects reduce as time progresses, although application of capsaicin outside the area of normal application at any stage can cause a reappearance of these effects. This application discomfort not infrequently leads to a failure in compliance (Box 12.1).

Occasionally sneezing can also occur, either in the patient or others living in close proximity, and usually occurs with over-application, drying of the cream on the skin, and the dust from this dried capsaicin being nasally inhaled. Caution should be used with capsaicin application to avoid application to moist areas (as this often exacerbates the discomfort associated with application) and that it is not accidentally applied to others, as in the case of a mother using the cream and then attending to a baby or child.

12.1.4 Tricyclic antidepressants

It is well accepted that oral tricyclic antidepressants can reduce neuropathic pain. This effect is achieved by virtue of a number of their modes of action:

- augmenting descending bulbo-spinal serotonergic inhibition
- augmenting descending bulbo-spinal noradrenergic inhibition
- an effect on NMDA (N-methyl D-aspartate) receptors
- an effect on opioid receptors
- sodium channel-blocking effects
- adenosine receptor-blocking effects.

We know that adenosine receptors, sodium channels, and opioid receptors have a peripheral, as well as central, representation, and therefore their analgesic effect may be peripheral as well as central. Both animal and human studies confirm that topical application of tricyclic antidepressants can reduce neuropathic pain and that this effect is locally generated and not caused by systemic absorption. Time to effect is two to four weeks and side-effects are rare, providing application volumes and area of application are not excessive. Commercially, the tricyclic antidepressant doxepin is available as a 5% cream.

12.1.5 **Clonidine**

Clonidine, an α_2-adrenoreceptor agonist, is available in a patch formulation to enable transdermal administration. However, patches may not be readily available in the UK. Two distinct effects can be achieved with transdermal clonidine. Firstly, a systemic effect which can alleviate neuropathic pain in a subset of patients with, for example, painful diabetic neuropathy. Secondly, it can reduce allodynia by a local action in some patients with sympathetically maintained pain.

12.2 **Oral agents**

12.2.1 **Mexiletine**

This oral, lidocaine-like, sodium channel-blocking anti-arrhythmic agent has been shown to have some effect in some patients with neuropathic pain. It has a narrow therapeutic index so use of effective dosages of mexiletine is not infrequently complicated by side-effects such as gastrointestinal upset and sedation.

12.2.2 **Baclofen**

Baclofen, a gamma amino butyric acid-B (GABA$_B$) agonist, is conventionally used as a skeletal muscle relaxant. However, it has been shown to reduce the pain associated with trigeminal neuralgia which is typified by intermittent flare-ups. Because of its fairly rapid onset of action, it can be used as an analgesic during these flare-ups. In most cases it is well tolerated and can be used with a starting dose of 10mg 3 times daily (decreased in the young, elderly, and infirm), increased up to a total of 60mg daily, if required.

12.2.3 **Tizanidine**

Again conventionally used as a skeletal muscle relaxant, tizanidine acts as an α_2-adrenoreceptor agonist. By virtue of this effect it can reduce neuropathic pain. Its principal side-effect is somnolence and therefore its use is particularly contemplated in the patient with neuropathic pain with secondary muscle spasm. The greater proportion of the daily dose is given at night to aid sleep.

12.2.4 **Cannabinoids**

Cannabinoids act both peripherally, via agonism at the specific cannabinoid receptors CB_1 and CB_2, and centrally. Much interest has focused on their use both as analgesics in neuropathic pain and as muscle relaxants. However, analysis of studies that examine the effect of the cannabinoids suggests that their analgesic effect in neuropathic pain is not as great as was initially suggested.

12.2.5 **5HT$_3$ antagonists**

The $5HT_3$ antagonist drugs are well established in the treatment of nausea and vomiting. They are now known to specifically block the neurokinin-1 (NK_1) expressing neurons in the dorsal horn of the spinal cord. These NK_1 expressing neurons are an important link in the spino-bulbo-cerebral transmission of pain signals and influence the descending control of dorsal horn function (see Chapter 2).

Use of a $5HT_3$ antagonist can therefore reduce certain types of pain and this includes neuropathic pain. They have a relatively benign side-effect profile with constipation and headache being the principal side-effects associated with sustained use. Members of the class include ondansetron, granisetron, dolasetron, and tropisetron.

12.2.6 **Cholecystokinin antagonists**

Cholecystokinin (CCK), originally described as a gut peptide, is now known to have central nervous system as well as gastrointestinal tract representation. The levels of this peptide in the central nervous system are increased by neural injury and sustained use of opioids, and it acts as an anti-opioid peptide. In animal pain models, administration of a CCK antagonist can not only enhance opioid-derived anti-nociception but also prevent and reverse established anti-nociceptive tolerance. To date, the human evidence merely suggests that the CCK antagonist proglumide enhances opioid-derived pain relief, with the question of its effects on opioid analgesic tolerance being unanswered.

12.2.7 **L-carnitine**

L-carnitine is synthesized in vivo from the amino acids lysine and methionine and has a role in transporting fatty acids from the cytosol to the mitochondria. In some countries it is sold as a nutritional supplement to which a number of benefits are attributed, including weight loss and reduction in depression.

Recent evidence has shown that carnitine has an effect on the expression of metabotropic glutamate receptors in lamina II, III and IV of the spinal cord and cerebral cortex. Human evidence suggests that treatment with L-carnitine can reduce neuropathic pain, and in particular that which complicates cancer chemotherapy, HIV infection and diabetes mellitus.

12.3 **Parenteral agents**

12.3.1 **Need for parenteral agents**

While long-term pharmacological therapy of neuropathic pain is best achieved by use of topical or oral preparations, there are occasions when parenteral administration of medication is desirable:

- when the oral route of administration is unavailable (for example when severe vomiting is taking place)
- when a rapid titration of drug is needed during acute flare-ups of neuropathic pain
- when oral therapy is insufficient on its own to reduce acute pain
- when, as with intravenous lidocaine, phenytoin, and fosphenytoin, the duration of analgesic effect of the drug far outlives the plasma half-life of the drug.

12.3.2 **Lidocaine**

For over 50 years it has been known that the intravenous (IV) infusion of local anaesthetics can be associated with pain relief in a wide variety of pain conditions, including neuropathic pain. Since the introduction of lidocaine this effect has been confirmed on numerous occasions with this drug.

Both animal experimentation and human use suggests that the pain-relieving effect that can be apparent after IV lidocaine infusion can be of significantly greater duration than the half-life of the drug. Indeed, weeks of pain relief can follow IV lidocaine infusion. Despite the fear of potential cardiovascular side-effects, cardiac arrhythmia and evidence of any negative inotropic effect are very uncommon.

A number of unanswered questions remain about IV lidocaine use:

- the optimal dose administered
- the optimal infusion period
- whether a single infusion or repeated infusions achieve maximum effect
- the role of a test infusion of lidocaine at a lower dose than a formal infusion
- whether a positive response to IV lidocaine actually confirms that oral mexiletine has a greater chance of achieving pain relief.

Despite these questions, there is no doubt that IV lidocaine infusion represents a useful treatment of neuropathic pain. When it is effective, patients can reduce their concomitant analgesic consumption as well as potentially reducing other agents, such as tricyclic antidepressants and antiepileptic drugs whose use is frequently associated with side-effects such as somnolence, weight gain, and effects on cognitive processes.

12.3.3 **Phenytoin**

It is of no surprise that the antiepileptic drug phenytoin, known to have anti-neuropathic pain effects when used orally, can also reduce such pain when given parenterally (see also Chapter 11). However, caution with IV phenytoin use is needed as the parenteral formulations contain highly alkaline substances, and so any extravasation of the infused phenytoin can cause skin necrosis.

12.3.4 **Fosphenytoin**

Fosphenytoin is a water-soluble, ester pro-drug of phenytoin with a near normal pH. Consequently, the danger of skin necrosis is significantly less than with phenytoin. It shares the analgesic effect of phenytoin and as such is a safer, if more expensive, alternative to parenteral phenytoin.

12.3.5 **5HT$_3$ antagonists**

As mentioned above, the 5HT$_3$ antagonists can reduce pain associated with a variety of pain conditions, including that of neuropathic origin. By virtue of their lack of sedating effects and their general safety profile, IV 5HT$_3$ antagonists can be usefully administered when a rapid resolution of neuropathic pain is required.

12.3.6 **Adenosine**

Adenosine receptors have both peripheral and central nervous system representation and animal work suggests that these receptors have a function in nociceptive transmission. Isolated human reports suggest that IV infusion of adenosine can achieve sustained pain relief in some patients with refractory neuropathic pain.

12.4 **Using other pharmacological approaches in practice**

Not all patients with neuropathic pain can be successfully treated with tricyclics, antiepileptics, or opioids. In further patients intolerable side-effects are apparent after use of drugs in these classes. It is therefore important to have alternatives. With some of the options listed in this chapter, a wealth of experience with their use exists. In others, such as the 5HT$_3$ antagonists and CCK antagonists, only time will tell if their use becomes commonplace in neuropathic pain management.

When formulating a treatment plan for the patient with neuropathic pain there is no such thing as the 'best' option. Rather, a range of alternatives will exist that all have the potential for producing pain relief, but none of which will offer a therapeutic guarantee. Some patients will elect to try the simple topical preparations first. Usually they lack the potential for serious adverse effects and yet not infrequently produce pain relief. At the other end of the spectrum, acute and serious flare-ups of pain require immediately-acting agents. The existence of parenteral lidocaine, fosphenytoin, and $5HT_3$ antagonists may remove the need to utilize immediate-release opioids with all their attendant side-effects.

Table 12.1 Dosing regimens for local anaesthetics and other co-analgesics			
Drug	Dose	Dose interval	Time to effect
Topical			
Lidocaine	5% patch	1 patch daily	days
Capsaicin	0.075% cream	4 times daily	2–4 weeks
Doxepin	5% cream	4 times daily	2 weeks
Oral			
Baclofen	10–20mg	3 times daily	days
Tizanidine	4–8mg	3 times daily	days
Mexiletine	50–150mg	4 times daily	days
Ondansetron	4mg	3 times daily	Hours
L-carnitine	500mg	Twice daily	days
Parenteral			
Lidocaine IV	500–1000mg	over 24 hours	immediate to 1 week
Phenytoin IV	600mg	over 24 hours	hours
Fosphenytoin IM	500PE*	once only	hours
Fosphenytoin IV	1000PE*	over 24 hours	hours
Ondansetron IV	8mg	once only	hours

* 1.5mg of fosphenytoin is equivalent to 1mg PE (phenytoin sodium equivalent).

IV = intravenous, IM = intramuscular.

Mexiletine may not be readily available in UK.

Cholecystokinin antagonists and cannabinoids not covered as currently commercially unavailable in UK.

Some of these regimens are unlicensed uses of drugs.

Key references

Flatters S.J., Xiao W.H., Bennett G.J. (2006). Acetyl-L-carnitine prevents and reduces paclitaxel-induced painful peripheral neuropathy. *Neurosci Lett*, **397**, 219–23.

McCleane, G.J. (2004). Cholecystokinin antagonists: a new way to improve analgesia from old analgesics? *Curr. Pharm. Des*, **10**, 303–14.

McCleane G.J. (2008). Topical Analgesic Agents. *Clin Geriatr Med*, **24**, 299–312.

McCleane GJ. (2008). *Pain management: expanding the pharmacological options*. Wiley-Blackwell, Oxford.

McCleane GJ. (2007). Intravenous lidocaine: an outdated or underutilized treatment for pain? *J Palliat Med*, **10**, 798–805.

McCleane GJ. (2008). Antidepressants as analgesics. *CNS Drugs*, **22**, 139–56.

Chapter 13

Ketamine and other NMDA receptor antagonists

Marie Fallon, Cameron Fergus and
Barry J.A. Laird

Key points

- Ketamine is a non-competitive N-methyl D-aspartate (NMDA) receptor antagonist and is most effective in pain states where hyper-excitability is established
- Ketamine undergoes first-pass metabolism to norketamine, which is a more potent analgesic than ketamine. This can explain why oral ketamine is more potent than parenteral ketamine
- There is much clinical experience supporting use of ketamine in neuropathic pain states but the evidence base is not well established
- Dextromethorphan is an alternative NMDA receptor antagonist and has been combined with morphine in some successful clinical trials
- It is likely that more selective NMDA receptor subtype antagonists will be identified and developed in the future.

13.1 Ketamine pharmacology

13.1.1 Background

Ketamine is a dissociative anaesthetic agent which was developed in the 1960s. At sub-analgesic doses, ketamine is a potent analgesic, but does not cause respiratory depression or clinically significant cardiovascular stimulation. More recently, it has been used in sub-anaesthetic doses for neuropathic pain of multiple aetiologies, for peri and post-operative analgesia, as well as for complex and refractory cancer pain, often in addition to opioids. Although there are relatively few randomized controlled trials of its use, there is a growing body of evidence for its effectiveness in the management of both malignant and non-malignant neuropathic pain.

13.1.2 **Pharmacodynamics**

The mode of action of ketamine is through non-competitive antagonism of the N-methyl-D-aspartate (NMDA) receptor gated calcium channel, located in the spinal cord (see Chapter 2). The NMDA receptor is not usually active under normal physiological conditions however in some pain states, such as neuropathic pain, the excitatory neurotransmitter glutamate is released which is an NMDA agonist and causes receptor activation. Activation of the NMDA receptor is a contributor to the development of 'wind-up' which results in central sensitization and opioid tolerance. Ketamine interacts with the NMDA receptor at the phencyclidine binding site, significantly inhibiting the receptor activity. This occurs only after the channel has been opened i.e. in active pain states. (See Figure 2.2, Chapter 2).

The effectiveness of ketamine is partially due to a wind down phenomenon at the NMDA receptor, resetting the pain transmission pathway. In other words, it is most effective in pain states, where hyper-excitability has been established.

13.1.3 **Pharmacokinetics**

Ketamine is both water and lipid soluble. It is metabolized by the liver into several metabolites, the most important of which is norketamine. Norketamine has a lower *anaesthetic* potency than ketamine but has greater *analgesic* potency. When ketamine is administered orally it undergoes first pass metabolism to norketamine, resulting in greater concentrations of norketamine than when administered parenterally. Norketamine subsequently undergoes hydroxylation and conjugation before being excreted renally. Doses of ketamine do not need to be altered in renal failure.

13.1.4 **Side-effects**

In addition to the NMDA receptor, ketamine interacts with opioid and muscarinic receptors, sodium and potassium channels, and inhibits serotonin and dopamine re-uptake. This activity at multiple receptors may be the basis of the unpleasant psychomimetic side-effects of ketamine. Side-effects include confusion, dysphoria, vivid dreams and hallucinations. Other side-effects include hypertension and tachycardia. The psychomimetic side-effects can be reduced or even prevented by the concomitant administration of haloperidol (2–4mg/day PO).

13.1.5 **Preparations**

Commercially available ketamine exists as a racemic mixture of its two stereoisomers: R(–) and S(+). S(+) ketamine is 3 to 4 times more potent as an analgesic than R(–) ketamine. S(+) ketamine also has fewer psychomimetic side-effects than R(–) ketamine when given in equianalgesic doses, as they both interact to the same extent with cholinergic receptors. Although S(+) ketamine is being increasingly studied, standard racemic ketamine is used most commonly and the majority of evidence exists for this. Ketamine is usually given orally or parenterally (most often intravenously or subcutaneously for chronic pain) but can also be given by the spinal or rectal route. There are also reports of its use topically (as 0.5% ketamine cream) and as an intranasal spray.

13.2 Clinical uses of ketamine

13.2.1 Peri-operative pain

Many studies have examined the role of ketamine in addition to opioid-analgesia in the peri-operative setting. A systematic review of randomized trials examining ketamine as an adjuvant analgesic failed to show a clear benefit of ketamine as a useful component of peri-operative analgesia. Furthermore, adjuvant ketamine does not offer any benefit over patient-controlled analgesia.

13.2.2 Peripheral neuropathic pain

Post herpetic neuralgia—Controlled trials have shown beneficial effects of intravenous ketamine for post herpetic neuralgia. One placebo-controlled study showed that intravenous ketamine improved pain, reduced allodynia and hyperpathia in post herpetic neuralgia, and numerous case reports support this.

Peripheral neuropathy—Ketamine is a useful adjuvant analgesic when other neuropathic agents have been ineffective. One trial examining ketamine in peripheral neuropathic pain of traumatic origin showed it to have a beneficial effect. Pain scores were reduced significantly compared to placebo, however the authors commented that side-effects of ketamine may limit its usefulness.

13.2.3 Central neuropathic pain

Ketamine has been examined in patients with central dysaesthesia pain after spinal cord injury. Ketamine reduced both continuous and evoked pain, but did not affect thermal sensitivity. Dysaesthesia pain after spinal cord injury may be dependent on the activation of central NMDA receptors and that ketamine may have a role in the treatment of this pain state.

13.2.4 Ischaemic pain

Ischaemic rest pain secondary to arteriosclerosis is thought to have both nociceptive and neuropathic elements and may be only partially opioid responsive. A double blind randomized controlled trial that compared regular opioids plus placebo with regular opioids plus ketamine showed a statistically significant improvement in pain relief, general activity and enjoyment of life, in the group treated with ketamine.

13.2.5 **Cancer pain**

The World Health Organization regards ketamine as an essential drug for refractory cancer pain. Unfortunately, there is a dearth of good quality, randomized, controlled trials of ketamine in cancer pain to provide a solid evidence base for its use. Four clinical trials were identified as part of a recent Cochrane review, however 2 of these were excluded because of inappropriate study design. The 2 accepted trials concluded that ketamine improves the effectiveness of morphine in the treatment of cancer pain. One trial compared ketamine 0.25 mg/kg and 0.5mg/kg intravenous bolus with placebo in 10 cancer patients with neuropathic pain that was unrelieved by morphine. Ketamine significantly reduced the pain intensity in almost all patients at both doses, with the effect being more marked at the higher dose. Psychomimetic side-effects were reported in 6 out of 10 patients and these were treated with diazepam.

The second included trial compared intrathecal morphine alone, with intrathecal morphine plus ketamine, in 20 patients with cancer neuropathic pain. The study suggested that ketamine enhanced the analgesic effect of morphine and no serious side-effects were reported in this study.

The Cochrane review of ketamine in cancer pain concluded that there was insufficient data to enable any evidence-based conclusions about the benefits and harms of adjuvant ketamine alongside opioid therapy. There are however many case reports and open label trials, describing the use of ketamine in combination with opioids in cancer pain. Many of these reports describe dramatic relief of pain in patients with refractory cancer pain. In most cases, the ketamine was used in addition to opioids, with treatment duration of between 4 hours and 1 year. Doses ranged from 1mg/kg/day by subcutaneous infusion to 600mg/day intravenously. Side-effects, including sedation and hallucinations, were generally not reported as being severe.

13.2.6 **Ketamine in children**

Studies of ketamine in children are limited. One randomized controlled trial showed that post-operative ketamine did not have an opioid sparing effect and had a high incidence of hallucinogenic side-effects. Ketamine has also been used as a pre-medication for painful procedures such as bone marrow aspiration and lumbar puncture in children. It has been reported as providing good analgesia with faster recovery time and fewer side effects than alternatives.

There are individual case reports of ketamine being, used in paediatric patients with cancer pain. One patient was a 2-year-old girl with severe pain from a metastatic neuroblastoma who was treated successfully with intravenous ketamine after an unsuccessful trial of methadone. Methadone had caused unacceptable side-effects including respiratory depression and sedation. Pain control was reasonable with ketamine and there was improvement in quality of life.

13.3 **Practical considerations**

13.3.1 **Patient selection**

Clinical experience with ketamine is extensive, principally within the palliative care community, but also within chronic pain clinics. However, research evidence in support of various practices is more limited. Clinicians familiar with ketamine usually suggest that it is used for neuropathic pain, which has not responded to standard treatment such as tricyclic antidepressants and anticonvulsants. It also has a place in cancer pain which is poorly or not responsive to opioids. Chronic pain states with features of central wind-up (allodynia, hyperalgesia, hyperpathia) in combination with poor opioid responsiveness, will usually trigger a trial of ketamine.

Ketamine is contraindicated in patients with raised intracranial pressure, uncontrolled hypertension, psychosis and epilepsy. It should be used with caution in patients with a history of cardiac failure or cerebrovascular disease. It may affect the hepatic metabolism of theophylline and levothyroxine. Monitoring of blood pressure and pulse is recommended when starting or increasing ketamine, see Table 13.1.

13.3.2 **Oral administration**

When ketamine is used orally, it is subject to extensive first pass metabolism, resulting in a bioavailability of between 15–30%. Nevertheless oral ketamine has been shown to have analgesic benefit when administered orally on a regular basis. This may be due in part to the production of the potent metabolite norketamine. A starting oral

Table 13.1 Ketamine in practice	
	Clinical management
Contraindications	
Uncontrolled hypertension	
Raised intracranial pressure	
Psychosis	
Epilepsy	
Cautions	
Cardiac failure	Monitor blood pressure and pulse
Cerebrovascular disease	
Adverse effects	
Psychomimetic (confusion, hallucinations, dysphoria)	Reduce dose, consider haloperidol or benzodiazepine

dose of 10mg 4 times daily is suggested, increasing in 5–10mg increments daily until a response is achieved, Table 13.2. The usual oral dose range is 10–60mg four times daily although there are reports of higher doses (up to 100mg qds) being used. A parenteral formulation (10mg/ml) can be used orally but is extremely bitter—the taste can be masked with juice. There is now an unlicensed oral preparation (50mg/5ml) available in the United Kingdom. This can be obtained by special order from Cardinal Health Martindale Pharma (see useful addresses).

13.3.3 **Parenteral administration**

Ketamine can be administered by either subcutaneous or intravenous infusion. Some clinicians administer the first dose of ketamine intravenously to assess response and monitor for side-effects. The optimum dose is not clear and varies depending on the route, Table 13.2. In all cases, ketamine should be commenced at a low dose and titrated as per response and side-effects. Some specialists advise a reduction of regular opioid dose by 33–50% at the start of ketamine treatment, or a switch to a short acting opioid. The usual parenteral dose range is 50–600mg/day, but doses of up to 2400mg/day have been reported.

When used parenterally, ketamine should be diluted with 0.9% saline and prepared daily. When being administered subcutaneously, the addition of 1mg dexamethasone to the syringe driver and daily rotation of the site may prevent subcutaneous inflammation. Concomitant use of haloperidol or a benzodiazepine may be necessary to reduce the risk of psychomimetic side-effects, see Table 13.3. Once pain has stabilized with ketamine, it may be continued for some time. There are reports of its use subcutaneously for over 1 year.

Table 13.2 Ketamine dosing schedules			
Route	Starting doses	Increments	Usual dose range
Oral (50 mg/ml solution)	10 mg qds	5–10 mg per dose (20–40 mg daily)	10–100 mg qds
Subcutaneous infusion (dilute in normal saline) Continuous Burst	50–150 mg/day 50–150 mg/day	50–100 mg daily 100 mg daily	50–600 mg/day 100–500 mg/day and between 3 and 5 doses only
Intravenous infusion (dilute in 500mls normal saline)	30–50mg over 4 hours	Increase by 30% if poor response	

	Table 13.3 Parenteral administration—Clinical Considerations
Side-effects	Be vigilant for psycho-mimetic side-effects Consider prophylactic haloperidol (1.5mg PO or 2mg IV) to counteract these.
Monitoring	Blood pressure, pulse, sedation and levels of pain—should be checked every 15 minutes during the first hour of intravenous/subcutaneous infusion. Stop if sedation, change in systolic BP (increase or decrease of 20mmHg) or bradycardia or respiratory depression
Opioid Dose	Consider reduction in opioid dose of between 33–50% prior to commencing treatment. DO NOT USE IF EVIDENCE OF OPIOID TOXICITY

13.3.4 Conversion from parenteral to oral dosing

If there is a good response to parenteral administration of ketamine, conversion to the oral route may be attempted. However, the first pass effect means that the oral dose does not correlate to the subcutaneous dose, and can mean that oral ketamine is more potent than parenteral ketamine. Because of this, some clinicians now start treatment with oral ketamine and avoid the initial subcutaneous titration for those patients able to use the oral route. There are case reports of conversion from subcutaneous to oral where good analgesia was achieved with oral ketamine at doses of 30–40% of the previous parenteral dose.

13.3.5 Intranasal and sublingual administration

Ketamine has been shown to be effective for breakthrough pain resulting in analgesia after 10 minutes and lasting up to 1 hour. Preparations delivering a dose of 10mg were used. It has also been shown to have a similar bioavailability to oral administration when used sublingually. In cancer pain, sublingual ketamine has been shown to be effective as breakthrough analgesia in patients receiving intrathecal analgesia.

13.3.6 Burst ketamine

Ketamine has been used as a continuous subcutaneous infusion over a short duration (3 to 5 days) at doses titrated between 100–500mg/24 hours—so called 'burst ketamine'. Although there are no placebo-controlled trials of its use in this way, response rates of up to 67% have been reported to the initial infusion, with sustained pain control for up to eight weeks after cessation of the ketamine.

13.4 **Other NMDA receptor antagonists**

13.4.1 **Magnesium**

Magnesium acts as an NMDA receptor antagonist and under normal physiological conditions it blocks the NMDA receptor. Magnesium sulphate has been used with benefit in animal models of neuropathic pain, and in treating migraine and post-operative pain in human studies. One of the advantages of magnesium over ketamine is that it has fewer side-effects. There is some evidence that intravenous magnesium sulphate may be an effective analgesic in patients with post-herpetic neuralgia. Of particular note is that it appears to be safe and well tolerated.

Magnesium sulphate has also been used for the treatment of neuropathic pain due to brachial or lumbosacral plexus infiltration by cancer. Doses of 500mg and 1g were used with benefit and with minimal side-effects. Due to a lack of controlled studies, the role of magnesium in the treatment of neuropathic pain has not been proven.

13.4.2 **Dizocilpine (MK-801)**

This is a non-competitive antagonist of the NMDA receptor which binds very strongly to the NMDA receptor. Unfortunately it has marked psychomimetic side-effects and this limits its use to animal models.

13.4.3 **Dextromethorphan**

Dextromethorphan has been shown to have NMDA receptor antagonist activity in experimental settings. It was introduced in the 1950s as an alternative opioid to morphine. Its main use in the United Kingdom is as an antitussive. As such, it is an ingredient in low doses in many over the counter cough preparations. Clinical trials of its use for non-cancer pain have produced variable results. One study in cancer pain found that dextromethorphan was ineffective.

Morphidex, a 1:1 combination of morphine and dextromethorphan has been studied in the United States, with disappointing results overall. In those trials of Morphidex with positive results, equianalgesic benefit was found at significantly lower morphine doses.

It has also been suggested that a good response to a small dose (0.1mg/kg) of intravenous ketamine is a useful predictor of the likelihood of response to oral dextromethorphan. At present, therefore, the role of dextromethorphan as an adjuvant treatment for neuropathic pain remains unclear. Although dextromethorphan (and perhaps magnesium) may have a role to play in the future management of neuropathic and difficult cancer pain, it is likely that more selective NMDA subtype antagonists will be identified and developed.

Useful Addresses

Ketamine—oral liquid—available from
Cardinal Health Martindale Products
www.martindalepharma.co.uk
Tel: 0800 137 627
Fax: 0800 393 360

Key References

Bell R., Eccleston C., Kalso E. (2003). Ketamine as an adjuvant to opioids for cancer pain. *Cochrane Database Syst Rev*(1): CD003351.

Carr D.B., Goudas L.C. *et al.* (2004). Safety and efficacy of intranasal ketamine in a mixed population with chronic pain. *Pain*, **110**(3), 762–4.

Chong C., Schug S. *et al.* (2006). Bioavailability of ketamine after oral or sublingual administration. *Pain Medicine*, **7**(5), 469.

Crosby V., Wilcock A. *et al.* (2000). The safety and efficacy of a single dose (500 mg or 1 g) of intravenous magnesium sulfate in neuropathic pain poorly responsive to strong opioid analgesics in patients with cancer. *J Pain Symptom Man*, **19**(1), 35–9.

Dix P., Martindale S. *et al.* (2003). Double-blind randomized placebo-controlled trial of the effect of ketamine on postoperative morphine consumption in children following appendicectomy. *Paediatr Anaesth*, **13**(5), 422–6.

Elia N. and Tramer M.R. (2005). Ketamine and postoperative pain—a quantitative systematic review of randomised trials. *Pain*, **113**(1–2), 61–70.

Fitzgibbon E.J., Hall P. *et al.* (2002). Low dose ketamine as an analgesic adjuvant in difficult pain syndromes: a strategy for conversion from parenteral to oral ketamine. *J Pain Symptom Man*, **23**(2), 165–70.

Jackson, K., Ashby M. et al. (2001). 'Burst' ketamine for refractory cancer pain: an open-label audit of 39 patients. *J Pain Symptom Man*, **22**(4), 834–42.

Kvarnstrom A., Karlsten R. *et al.* (2003). The effectiveness of intravenous ketamine and lidocaine on peripheral neuropathic pain. *Acta Anaesthesiol Scand*, **47**(7), 868–77.

Mercadante S., Arcuri E. *et al.* (2005). Alternative treatments of breakthrough pain in patients receiving spinal analgesics for cancer pain. *J Pain Symptom Man*, **30**(5), 485–91.

Mercadante S., Arcuri E. *et al.* (2000). Analgesic effect of intravenous ketamine in cancer patients on morphine therapy: a randomized, controlled, double-blind, crossover, double-dose study. *J Pain Symptom Man*, **20**(4), 246–52.

Mitchell A.C., Fallon M.T. (2002). A single infusion of intravenous ketamine improves pain relief in patients with critical limb ischaemia: results of a double blind randomised controlled trial. *Pain*, **97**(3), 275–81.

Subramaniam K., Subramaniam B. *et al.* (2004). Ketamine as adjuvant analgesic to opioids: a quantitative and qualitative systematic review. *Anesth Analg*, **99**(2), 482–95, table of contents.

Visser E., and Schug S.A. (2006). The role of ketamine in pain management. *Biomed Pharmacother*, **60**(7), 341–8.

Chapter 14

Opioids

Michael I. Bennett

Key points

- Opioid receptor structure and function can be altered in neuropathic pain states, leading to reduced sensitivity to opioids
- Opioids were thought to be ineffective for neuropathic pain but substantial evidence exists to demonstrate analgesic efficacy, in some cases superior to more commonly used co-analgesics
- The most convincing evidence supports use of morphine, oxycodone, and tramadol in neuropathic pain
- Methadone, buprenorphine, and fentanyl may have a role but are supported by less convincing evidence, though the evidence base is growing rapidly
- Opioids should be used with caution in chronic pain management because of unknown long-term effects and risk of misuse. Adherence to local protocols and guidelines is recommended.

14.1 Opioids, opioid receptors, and neuropathic pain

14.1.1 History of opioids in neuropathic pain

The term 'opioid' includes naturally occurring, semi-synthetic, and synthetic drugs which, like morphine, combine with opioid receptors to produce their effects. An 'opiate' is a drug derived from the opium poppy, such as morphine and codeine.

The place of opioids in the management of neuropathic pain has been controversial until relatively recently. Clinical observations in the 1970s and 1980s of patients with nociceptive and neuropathic pain diagnoses who were given single doses of opioids suggested that neuropathic pain was resistant to opioids. These studies were often small, non-randomized, and uncontrolled, though their conclusions were readily taken up by some clinicians. By the 1990s, observational and controlled studies began to emerge that demonstrated dose responsiveness to opioids in patients with neuropathic pain. Although patients with nociceptive pain experienced greater pain relief, it was clear that neuropathic pain appears to confer reduced sensitivity to opioids, rather than resistance. Over the last 10 years, much more consistent evidence has emerged to support the use of opioids as a class (as well as individual drugs) in the treatment of neuropathic pain.

14.1.2 Types of opioid receptors

There are at least three types of opioid receptor that mediate analgesia: μ (mu), κ (kappa), and δ (delta) (Table 14.1). A fourth receptor, called nociceptin orphanin FQ peptide (NOP), shares the structural characteristics of other opioid receptors but has low affinity for opioid agonists and antagonists. In clinical practice, therapeutic opioids are largely active at μ receptors and their effects are antagonized by naloxone. Recent research in animal models suggests that a novel form of the μ receptor may exist. This receptor binds diamorphine (heroin) and morphine-6-glucuronide (M6G) with high affinity, but has no interaction with morphine.

14.1.3 Opioid receptor activation

Opioid receptors are G-protein-coupled receptors and are found throughout the spinal cord and in many areas of the brain. Opioid receptors are located pre-synaptically on primary afferent neurons within the dorsal horn of the spinal cord. Once activated, they inhibit glutamate release and hence inhibit transmission of nociceptive stimuli from C and Aδ fibres.

Activated opioid receptors may also reduce gamma amino butyric acid (GABA) release within the peri-aquaductal grey (PAG), an area of the midbrain involved in the central control of nociceptive transmission. GABA is the main inhibitory transmitter in the brain and acts to reduce or prevent anti-nociceptive outflow descending to the spinal cord from the PAG. Thus the additional effect of opioids is to block GABA and therefore boost the descending inhibitory control pathway, reducing pain transmission.

Table 14.1 Opioid receptors	
Opioid receptor subtype	Effect of agonist
Mu	Analgesia, respiratory depression, reduced gastrointestinal motility, hypotension
Kappa	Analgesia, sedation, psychomimetic effects, some respiratory depression
Delta	Analgesia, respiratory depression
NOP	Little evidence of clinical effect of agonist or antagonist

14.1.4 **Opioid receptors in neuropathic pain**

Laboratory work has provided a number of explanations why neuropathic pain exhibits reduced sensitivity to opioids. This includes genetic variation in receptor sensitivity and in particular the influence of genetic polymorphisms. These are minor changes in the amino acid sequencing of receptors and their associated proteins that impact on opioid binding. Additional factors include loss of opioid receptors on pre-synaptic spinal terminals and up-regulation of the neuromodulator cholecystokinin (CCK) which antagonizes opioid effects. Other evidence suggests that neuropathic pain causes opioid receptors themselves to become un-coupled from the G-proteins that they usually activate, resulting in lack of activity even if a drug binds to the opioid receptor.

14.1.5 **Opioids and hypersensitivity**

Emerging evidence suggests that the clinical effects of opioids are mediated not only by their analgesic or anti-nociceptive activity (the ability to reduce pain signals), but also by their ability to inhibit excitation or 'wind-up' processes (see also Chapter 2). Some opioids that are pure μ agonists are thought to induce excitation when used in large doses and there is some clinical evidence to support this. In contrast, opioids that have antagonist activity at certain receptors may inhibit processes that lead to excitation, e.g. methadone and buprenorphine. Evidence to support this is reviewed under each drug.

14.2 **Morphine**

14.2.1 **Pharmacology**

Morphine is a natural derivative of the opium poppy and is the prototypical μ receptor agonist. It is readily absorbed after oral administration, mainly in the upper small bowel, and is metabolized in the liver and at other sites to morphine-3-glucuronide (M3G) and M6G. M6G is an active metabolite and is a more potent analgesic than morphine. Morphine and its glucuronides are renally excreted and so may accumulate with impaired renal function.

Morphine is available as oral normal-release and modified-release preparations, as well as injections. Normal-release oral preparations of morphine generally produce analgesic effects within one hour (oral solution is faster than tablets), with a plasma half-life of around 2 hours. Modified-release preparations are effective within 2 to 3 hours, with a plasma half-life of approximately 4 to 6 hours.

Table 14.2 Opioid activity at receptor sites

	Mu	Kappa	Delta	NOP	NMDA	Serotonergic	Noradrenergic
Morphine	+						
Oxycodone	+	+					
Fentanyl	++						
Tramadol	+					+	+
Methadone	+				−		
Buprenorphine	(+)	−	−				
Diamorphine	+						

+ = full agonist
(+) = partial agonist
− = antagonist

14.2.2 **Clinical studies**

Morphine was originally thought to improve mood alone, rather than pain, in patients with neuropathic pain. Single-dose and longer-term studies in patients with post-herpetic neuralgia, however, showed that morphine is as effective as intravenous (IV) lidocaine and oral tricyclic antidepressants, and all these treatments were significantly better than placebo. A well-designed study compared morphine, gabapentin, placebo, and combined morphine/gabapentin in a group of patients with post-herpetic neuralgia or diabetic neuropathy. This showed that morphine produced as good pain relief as gabapentin in these patients (in fact, slightly better—see Chapter 18 for more details).

In central neuropathic pain, morphine has also been shown to reduce brush-evoked allodynia compared to placebo in the short term, but was less successful in the longer term, at 1 year.

14.3 **Oxycodone**

14.3.1 **Pharmacology**

Oxycodone is a semi-synthetic opioid with many similarities to morphine. A potentially important difference is that oxycodone has activity at both μ and κ opioid receptors though the contribution of the latter to the clinical effects of oxycodone is disputed by some researchers. Activity at this additional site has been used to explain the effectiveness of oxycodone in neuropathic pain and a reduction in adverse cognitive effects compared to morphine (though possibly a higher incidence of constipation). Oxycodone has a high oral to parenteral availability and a twofold greater potency than morphine (i.e. 1mg oral oxycodone = 2mg oral morphine). It is metabolized to inactive substances.

Oxycodone is available as normal-release tablets and solution, and modified-release preparations, as well as injections. In the USA oxycodone is available in combination with paracetamol and has proved a very useful drug for both cancer and non-cancer chronic pain. Parenteral preparations allow continuity of analgesic effect for patients treated with oral oxycodone who are no longer able to take oral medicine, for example peri-operatively or in a palliative care context.

14.3.2 **Clinical studies**

Clinical studies of modified-release oxycodone have provided strong evidence of efficacy in the management of neuropathic pain. Two relatively small randomized controlled trials (RCTs) of less than 40 patients have been conducted in post-herpetic neuralgia and in diabetic neuropathy (though one used an active placebo to mimic side-effects). These studies showed significant improvements in the treatment arm compared to placebo, even though adverse effects were greater with treatment. Another larger RCT in diabetic neuropathy, conducted over 6 weeks, also showed a significant reduction in pain ratings compared to placebo.

In all these studies, ongoing and spontaneous pains were improved, and significant reductions in pain interference scores were noted, without changes in scores of mood. These data suggest that oxycodone can improve neuropathic pain and functioning and that these improvements are not brought about by changes in mood. Meta-analyses show that the number needed to treat (NNT) for oxycodone is 2.5. This means that one in every 2.5 (or 4 out of 10) patients with neuropathic pain treated with this drug will get around 50% reduction in their pain.

14.4 Fentanyl

14.4.1 **Pharmacology**

Fentanyl is a very potent synthetic opioid that is quickly metabolized to the inactive metabolite norfentanyl and excreted via the kidneys. It is approximately 100 times as potent as morphine (1mg fentanyl = 100mg morphine) and is safe to use in patients with renal impairment or renal failure, in contrast to morphine.

Fentanyl is highly lipophilic, meaning that it is readily absorbed into tissue containing fat and is therefore ideal for topical use. Fentanyl is available as transdermal patches that deliver a steady release of fentanyl into a subcutaneous depot over a three-day period. However, fentanyl clearance is slower in elderly patients and so sustained-release preparations should be used with caution in this population. It is also available as oral transmucosal fentanyl citrate lozenges and buccal tablets and absorption onto the buccal mucosa. These can provide rapid release of fentanyl and are often used to control cancer breakthrough pain, though there is no evidence to support their specific use in neuropathic pain.

14.4.2 **Clinical studies**

Studies in the late 1990s showed that single-dose IV fentanyl provided significantly better relief of neuropathic pain, compared to either diazepam or placebo, in patients with a variety of neuropathic pain diagnoses. Based on this success, the research group logically thought that continuation with fentanyl therapy, in the form of sustained-release transdermal patches, should be tested. In the open-label trial, the original patients did not do as well when followed up over a four-week period. Only a third felt some relief of their pain; the other two-thirds experienced no improvement or adverse effects leading to withdrawal. More recently, an open label study in 40 patients with mixed neuropathic pain conditions has shown that transdermal fentanyl was successful in reducing pain.

14.5 **Tramadol**

14.5.1 **Pharmacology**

Tramadol is often considered a weak opioid in contrast to the strong opioids morphine, oxycodone, and fentanyl. It is active at μ opioid receptors as well as enhancing central serotonergic and noradrenergic inhibition of pain. Although these additional actions are thought to enhance its analgesic effects, they may also be responsible for additional antimuscarinic adverse effects. Tramadol is around 5 to 8 times less potent than morphine (i.e. 50–80mg tramadol = 10mg morphine). Preparations are available as normal-release and modified-release tablets.

14.5.2 **Clinical studies**

Tramadol has been evaluated in separate RCTs of patients with post-herpetic neuralgia and diabetic neuropathy. These studies have provided a reasonable evidence base for demonstrating its effectiveness in neuropathic pain. A Cochrane review found that the NNT for tramadol is 3.5, meaning that 2 patients in 7 with neuropathic pain will get about 50% reduction in their pain with tramadol.

14.6 **Methadone**

14.6.1 **Pharmacology**

Methadone is a synthetic opioid and is well absorbed after oral administration. Its effects are largely mediated through μ opioid receptors but it exists as a racemic mixture. L-methadone produces opioid effects but D-methadone is active at NMDA receptors (see Chapters 2 and 13). Its average half-life is 24 hours, although this may vary between eight and 80 hours in different individuals, and there is a clear age-related increase in half-life. Methadone should be used with extreme caution, particularly in the elderly, because its unpredictable half-life means that accumulation may occur. This also means that its potency ratio to morphine has been difficult to establish. Best estimates suggest it is 5 to 10 times more potent than morphine with chronic administration (i.e. regular dosing with methadone 10mg = regular dosing with 50–100mg of morphine). It is metabolized to inactive substances.

14.6.2 **Clinical studies**

In neuropathic pain, methadone has been shown to have significantly better analgesic effects than placebo when given over a two-week period to patients with a mixture of neuropathic pain diagnoses. Whether methadone is superior to other opioids because of its NMDA receptor activity has yet to be demonstrated. Indeed, various studies have examined conversion ratios of morphine to methadone in patients with chronic pain. A higher ratio (signifying less methadone required for the same degree of pain relief, compared to morphine) was not seen in patients with neuropathic pain. This suggests that NMDA activity is minimal and that it is the μ agonist activity of methadone that results in the principal analgesic effect.

However, anecdotal reports exist describing the successful use of methadone in patients with severe cancer neuropathic pain previously treated with morphine. These patients had exhibited signs of excitation or hypersensitivity on large doses of morphine (generalized allodynia, myoclonus, increasing doses led to worse pain), but were well controlled on relatively low doses of methadone. Whether this success was due to NMDA antagonism or just a reduction in overall opioid dose is not clear.

14.7 Buprenorphine

14.7.1 Pharmacology

Buprenorphine is a partial μ agonist but has antagonist actions at κ and δ opioid receptors. It is available as sublingual tablets and more recently as transdermal patches that are similar in action to fentanyl patches. Buprenorphine is metabolized to inactive substances. Animal and volunteer studies suggest that buprenorphine has the highest antihyperalgesic effect of all opioids, i.e. it is most able to inhibit excitation.

14.7.2 Clinical studies

Clinical evidence supporting a role for buprenorphine in neuropathic pain is only just emerging and currently is not as strong as for some other opioids. Case series exist describing the effective use of buprenorphine in post-thoracotomy neuropathic pain and in cases where other opioids have failed to control pain dominated by neuropathic features. Further research is needed to examine whether the theoretical advantages of buprenorphine translate into clinical effectiveness.

14.8 Diamorphine

No specific evidence supports the use of diamorphine in neuropathic pain. This is probably because it is only available in a few countries, mainly the UK (and specifically not the USA where many drug studies are conducted), and has always been thought of as a pro-drug for morphine. The cloning of a novel μ receptor that is activated by diamorphine and M6G, and not morphine, may lead to new research on diamorphine in neuropathic pain.

Anecdotally (and in a palliative care setting), some patients with cancer neuropathic pain do experience greater analgesia with diamorphine via injection or subcutaneous infusion, than with oral morphine. This is often regarded as illogical or counter-intuitive, but could be explained by differences in opioid receptor expression and activity. Diamorphine is highly soluble and this allows large doses to be given in very small volumes.

14.9 Opioids in clinical practice

14.9.1 Need for caution

Although there is now a large body of evidence demonstrating the analgesic *efficacy* of opioids in neuropathic pain, a number of concerns exist about the *effectiveness* of opioids in clinical practice. These relate to well-described adverse effects that appear in the short term, fears about tolerance and addiction, and relatively unknown long-term, and potentially irreversible, effects of opioids. However, there is no doubt that opioids have a role in both cancer and non-cancer neuropathic pain. In the latter context, careful selection and adherence to local protocols, that may include patient contracts, may be necessary.

14.9.2 Common adverse effects

Common adverse effects that can appear relatively soon after initiating treatment with opioids include somnolence and other cognitive effects, nausea, and constipation (Table 14.3). Sedation is common when commencing morphine and after the dose has been increased. It usually wears off after 2 to 3 days at the same dose, and patients on stable doses of morphine can be allowed to drive. Hallucinations, confusion, and vivid dreams may necessitate a dose reduction or a change to an alternative opioid; alternatively they can be managed with a small dose of haloperidol (1.5–3mg) at night. Side-effects

Table 14.3 Opioid side-effects		
Side-effect	Generally dose related?	Management strategy
Dry mouth	No	Frequent mouth care, artificial saliva
Constipation	Probably not	Prophylactic laxative, e.g. co-danthramer
Nausea	Yes	Tends to wear off, regular meto clopramide if not
Sedation or confusion	Yes	Reduce dose by 30%, check renal function, may respond to change of opioid
Hallucinations	Yes	Reduce dose by 30%, consider haloperidol, may respond to change of opioid
Pruritus	No	May respond to change of opioid

should be discussed with patients before they decide to commence opioids. There is no evidence that patients on chronic opioids are cognitively impaired or are unable to drive safely. However, patients must be warned about driving when commencing opioids. They should be advised not to drive for one to two weeks after commencing treatment or increasing dose and that their insurance company may need to be informed of all medication that they are taking.

All opioids can cause nausea (30–50% of patients), vomiting (10% of patients), and constipation (around 80%). Constipation is usually greatest when commencing opioids. There is some evidence to support the concept that tolerance may develop to the constipating effects of opioids over time, and that a ceiling effect of opioid-induced constipation is reached relatively early. In other words, once established on opioids, patients may not be any more constipated if the dose is increased. All patients commenced on opioids should be prescribed softening and stimulant laxatives and have access to an antiemetic. Other well-recognized side-effects are dry mouth, itching, sweating, myoclonic jerks, and occasionally hypotension.

Respiratory depression is unusual but may occur in opioid-naive patients given a large dose of an opioid for acute pain, or due to a drug error or accumulation of opioid in the very elderly or its metabolites in renal failure. In chronic use, tolerance to the respiratory depressant effects occurs rapidly and provided the dose is titrated against the patient's pain, opioids can be used safely, even in patients with chronic lung disease. A physiological explanation for this is that the respiratory centre receives nociceptive input which counterbalances the respiratory potential of the opioid.

14.9.3 Fears about tolerance and addiction

Both professionals and patients have fears about the use of strong opioids, particularly morphine (Table 14.4). These fears are largely unfounded and with careful, knowledgeable use there are few problems. However, since these fears are common and may lead to poor pain management, the professional will need to discuss these issues with the patient when commencing strong opioids.

Table 14.4 Fears about opioid use	
Professional's fears	**Patient's fears**
Addiction	Addiction
Respiratory depression	Side-effects
Excess sedation	Tolerance
Confusion	Decreased options for future pain relief

Tolerance is the need for a higher dose to achieve the same pharmacological effect. There is no doubt (from experimental studies in acute pain) that tolerance to opioids can occur, possibly through down-regulation of opioid receptors after prolonged exposure to opioid agonists. The clinically relevant issue is to what extent this can be managed by careful patient selection, opioid switching (see Chapter 18), or alternative combinations of analgesics.

Patients with cancer-related pain often have an unfounded fear that if they start taking opioids, the drugs won't work later, when they really need it. An increase in analgesic requirement is usually due to an increase in pain due to advancing disease, rather than to tolerance.

Addiction does not occur when opioids are used carefully for the management of pain. If the cause of the pain is removed (e.g. by a nerve block or healing of an injury) then opioids can generally be reduced or withdrawn with no psychological problems. Occasionally there is a degree of *physical* dependence, with a physical withdrawal syndrome apparent upon withdrawal of the drug. This is characterized by fatigue, yawning, lacrimation, myalgia/arthralgia, and anxiety through to tachycardia, abdominal cramps, diarrhoea, nausea, and insomnia in more severe cases. However, when the opioid is withdrawn in staged decrements, this is easily managed.

Psychological dependence is a compulsion to continue to take the opioid because of the need for stimulation or because it relieves anxiety. Only a very small proportion of patients with chronic pain will develop psychological dependence. If there is drug-seeking behaviour or the apparent rapid development of tolerance to opioids in an otherwise stable pain (exclude disease progression or deterioration), clinicians should urgently review the patient and this may require the help of a specialist addiction service. Helpful guidelines on the use of opioids in patients with chronic non-cancer-related pain can be found on the British Pain Society's website (see Appendix 1).

14.9.4 **Long-term effects of opioids**

Many studies of opioids in chronic neuropathic pain are of relatively short duration—days to weeks. In clinical practice, commencing a patient on opioids may result in months or years of treatment and the long-term effects of opioids are relatively unknown. Current concerns relate to the long-term opioid effects on endocrine and immune systems. Specifically, infertility and suppressed immunity are potential consequences. Babies born of women who take long-term opioids may develop respiratory depression at birth and require specialist help.

Key references

Agarwal S., Polydefkis M., Block B., Haythornthwaite J., Raja S.N. (2007). Transdermal fentanyl reduces pain and improves functional activity in neuropathic pain states. *Pain Med*, **8**(7), 554–62.

Boureau, F., Legallicier, P., Marmar, K. (2003). Tramadol in post-herpetic neuralgia: a randomized, double-blind, placebo-controlled trial. *Pain*, **104**, 323–31.

Dellemijn, P.L., van Duijn, H., and Vanneste, J.A. (1998). Prolonged treatment with transdermal fentanyl in neuropathic pain. *J Pain Symptom Man*, **16**, 220–9.

Eisenberg E., McNicol E., Carr D.B. (2006). Opioids for neuropathic pain. *Cochrane Database Syst Rev*; 3:CD006146.

Gilron, I., Bailey, J.M., Dongsheng, T., Holden, R.R., Weaver, D.F., and Houlden, R.L. (2005). Morphine, gabapentin, or their combination for neuropathic pain. *N Engl J Med*, **352**, 1324–34.

Kalso E., Simpson K.H., Slappendel R., Dejonckheere J., Richarz U. (2007). Predicting long-term response to strong opioids in patients with low back pain: findings from a randomized, controlled trial of transdermal fentanyl and morphine. *BMC Med*, **5**, 39.

Koppert, W., Ihmsen, H., Korber, N., Wehrfritz, A., Sittl, R., Schmelz, M., et al. (2005). Different profiles of buprenorphine-induced analgesia and antihyperalgesia in a human pain model. *Pain*, **118**, 15–22.

Kress H.G. (2008). Clinical update on the pharmacology, efficacy and safety of transdermal buprenorphine. *Eur J Pain* **13**(3), 219–30.

Morley, J.S., Bridson, J., Nash, T., Miles, J.B., White, S., Makin, M.K. (2003). Low-dose methadone has an analgesic effect in neuropathic pain: a double-blind randomised controlled crossover trial. *Palliat Med*, **17**, 576–87.

Nielsen C.K., Ross F.B., Lotfipour S., Saini K.S., Edwards S.R., Smith M.T. (2007). Oxycodone and morphine have distinctly different pharmacological profiles: radioligand binding and behavioural studies in two rat models of neuropathic pain. *Pain*, **132**(3), 289–300.

Simonnet, G. (2005). Opioids: from analgesia to antihyperalgesia? *Pain*, **118**, 8–9.

Watson, C.P., Moulin, D., Watt-Watson, J., Gordon, A., Eisenhoffer, J. (2003). Controlled-release oxycodone relieves neuropathic pain: a randomized controlled trial in painful diabetic neuropathy. *Pain*, **105**, 71–8.

Chapter 15

Intrathecal drug delivery and neurolytic blocks

Karen H. Simpson and Iain Jones

Key points

- Intrathecal drug delivery (ITDD) allows drugs to be placed near to central receptors
- Drug side-effects may be reduced as small doses are required compared to with systemic administration
- External or internal ITDD systems are available
- ITDD requires careful patient selection and preparation
- Opioids, local anaesthetics, and clonidine are the most commonly used intrathecal drugs; ziconotide can be used as first line treatment
- Neurolytic blocks are usually used for neuropathic pain arising from cancer or peripheral vascular disease
- Coeliac plexus block for upper abdominal cancer pain or lumbar sympathectomy for ischaemic leg pain are very effective
- Intracerebroventricular drug delivery is possible for head pain usually due to cancer; but it is rarely used.

15.1 Intrathecal drug delivery

15.1.1 Background evidence

Intrathecal drug delivery (ITDD) allows drugs to be placed near to central receptors. Small drug doses are required compared to systemic administration; so drug side-effects may be reduced. ITDD was pioneered for cancer pain, and there is a systematic review that supports intrathecal opioid therapy that has not been adequately controlled by systemic treatment. For non-cancer pain there are several case series suggesting benefit of ITDD and one systematic review of the evidence for programmable ITDD for non-cancer pain. Pain intensity ratings seemed to remain fairly stable over the first year after ITDD implantation: data regarding changes after the first year were inconclusive. Success rates (proportions of patients with greater than 50% pain relief with patients lost to follow up considered failures) ranged from 38–56% at 6 months and from 30–44% at longer follow-up.

Further research is needed to evaluate more rigorously whether certain types of pain respond differentially to different intrathecal drugs. Among patients who were treated with opioids alone, those with neuropathic pain had a significantly lower success rate than did those with mechanical or mixed pain (89% vs. 100%). In a study that compared the efficacy and cost-effectiveness of ITDD with conventional therapy for pain from failed back surgery syndrome over five years, there was a 27% improvement in the ITDD groups' disability compared with 12% in the controls. The high initial costs of ITDD were recovered by 28 months and conventional therapy became relatively more expensive.

15.1.2 Practical considerations

Patient selection; Careful selection and screening offer the best chance of successful outcomes. For patients with cancer related pain the indications for ITDD are failed treatment with oral analgesics due to lack of efficacy or intolerable side effects and, for fully implanted programmable devices, a life expectancy of at least 3 months. Patients with neuropathic pain were thought to be poor candidates for ITDD; however recent studies have shown that opioids as well as local anaesthetics, clonidine and ziconotide can be effective in reducing refractory neuropathic pain. In general when considering ITDD for patients with non-cancer pain, patients are expected to have failed a range of therapies e.g. exercise, rehabilitation, psychological strategies, medication, nerve blocks, cognitive behavioural therapy and, in selected cases, spinal cord stimulation. Psychological factors are more likely to be relevant in long-term treatment of non-cancer pain, and therefore psychological evaluation is recommended for this group.

Patients with non-cancer pain usually have a longer life expectancy and thus longer requirement for long term pain relief than those with cancer. This may be relevant as opioid tolerance can occur, leading to dose escalation and possible dependence. Therefore additional contraindications in the non-cancer pain group may be important e.g. major psychiatric disorders, poor compliance, insufficient understanding of the therapy, lack of social support, drug and alcohol abuse and past drug seeking behaviours. ITDD should only be considered if simpler, safer, and more economical methods of analgesia have provided inadequate benefits. Patients must be carefully selected to ensure that ITDD is appropriate (Box 15.1).

Box 15.1 Indications and contraindications to ITDD

Indications

- Systemic analgesia effective but intolerable side-effects
- Good response to test dose or test infusion
- Favourable psychosocial evaluation
- Multidisciplinary team experienced with ITDD; on call service available
- Appropriate links to primary and secondary care teams.

Contraindications

- Patient refusal
- Head pain (often better managed by intracerebroventricular drug delivery)
- Inadequate analgesia or intolerable side-effects from IT testing
- Poor patient compliance with ITDD
- Systemic infection (care with diabetes, immune suppression, steroids and neutropenia)
- Localized infection in sites of potential surgery
- Non-correctable coagulopathy
- Raised intracranial pressure
- Impending spinal cord compression
- Allergy to intrathecal medication or implantable device components
- Lack of support services for ongoing care.

An intrathecal (IT) test dose of the proposed medication(s) may predict whether ITDD is indicated. There are differences in response to bolus injection and infusion, so testing requires careful assessment. Using the epidural route for testing may be unhelpful as some drugs do not cross the dura readily and dose equivalence is unclear. Regardless of the screening method it is important to place the drug at the spinal level of the origin of the pain. However, morphine is hydrophilic and moves readily through the CSF and so may cover a wider area. At least a 50% reduction in pain without intolerable side effects to the test drug is usually taken as a benchmark for a patient to be an appropriate candidate for ITDD.

ITDD must be performed under full asepsis with fluoroscopic guidance. General anaesthesia may be needed, especially in children or if pain prevents positioning of the patient. The main infection risk seems to correlate with the procedure duration, so it is important that experienced teams are involved. ITDD is a long-term commitment for the patient and the health care teams. It is invasive and there are risks of procedure, equipment-related, and drug-related complications that must be explained to patients and their carers (Table 15.1).

Table 15.1 Complications of ITDD Always check for causes not related to ITDD	
Complication	Management
Procedure related	
Post-spinal headache	Nurse supine, standard analgesia, IV fluids if emesis occurs, ?autologous epidural blood patch
Total spinal	Aggressive resuscitation
Bleeding	Clinical observation for cord/cauda equina compression, magnetic resonance imaging (MRI), alert surgeon early
Damage to cord/nerve roots	MRI early, surgical referral
Infection	Prevent infection - strict standard unit protocols, single dose of prophylactic antibiotics pre-implant, no evidence to support post-implant antibiotics
	Suspected infection - hospitalization, infection screen, microbiologist advice, aggressive anti-microbials
Superficial wound infection	Frequent observation, antibiotics
Pump pocket seroma	If infected, intravenous (IV) antibiotics, removal of the system usually required
Catheter/implant pocket infection	Remove system, IV antibiotics
Meningitis	Remove system, IV antibiotics
Epidural abscess	Whole spine MRI, alert surgeon, remove system, IV antibiotics

Table 15.1 Contd.

Complication	Management
Drug related—immediate	
Opioid	
Nausea and vomiting, urinary retention, pruritis, ventilatory depression, confusion	Antiemetics Intermittent catheterization Antihistamines, ondansetron Naloxone Review systemic and ITDD doses; change IT drugs
Ziconotide	
Nausea, vomiting, dizziness, blurred vision, memory impairment, depression, confusion, hallucinations, orthostatic hypotension	Reduce dose or stop infusion; consider slower dose titration
Local anaesthetic	
Numbness, urinary retention, orthostatic hypotension, motor block	Reduce dose
Clonidine	
Sedation, lethargy, hypotension, dry mouth, bowel disturbance	Reduce dose
Drug related—delayed	
Opioid	
Myoclonus, oedema or arthralgia, facial flushing or sweating, constipation, endocrine suppression	Change from opioids or use systemic benzodiazepine Change from opioids Systemic low dose clonidine Bowel care Monitor endocrine function, endocrine replacement treatments
Equipment related	
Allergy to equipment	May require removal of system; implantation testing may be needed
Catheter obstruction	Clear system under radiological screening; may need surgery
Catheter sheer, damage and/or spinal fluid leak	Manage headache; may need surgery
Catheter tip granuloma	MRI, surgical decompression, and removal of mass/catheter
Pump failure or over delivery; refill or programming error	Stop pump and manage drug effects; check pump; provide replacement drug therapy
Over dose	
Under dose	

15.1.3 **ITDD systems**

External systems are appropriate for patients with a relatively short life expectancy (<3 months) and for those who require larger volume spinal infusions. The procedure is simple; systems may be implanted under either local or general anaesthesia. Recovery after implant is usually quick. The catheter is tunnelled subcutaneously away from the spine, usually to the abdomen. The system has 2 antibacterial filters and must remain closed; boluses must be given from the pump if needed and never by opening the system and injecting. An external pump is used that has a capacity of at least 250 ml, can give very low volume infusions with precision, is easy to programme and is portable.

Fully implantable pumps may be gas driven; these deliver medication at a fixed rate. Dose changes are made by refilling the device with different drug concentrations; these are only useful in patients on predictable and stable doses. ITDD devices may be battery driven and these are programmed via non-invasive telemetry (Figure 15.1); some of the programmable pumps allow patients to deliver boluses

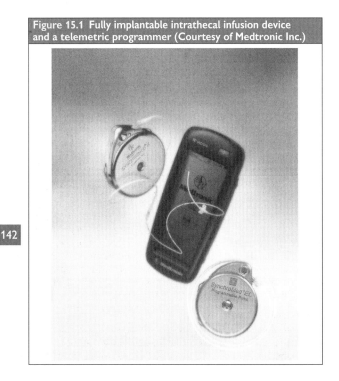

Figure 15.1 Fully implantable intrathecal infusion device and a telemetric programmer (Courtesy of Medtronic Inc.)

using a patient held telemetry device. The 10–50ml pump is implanted into a subcutaneous pocket in the abdominal wall, often under general anaesthesia. It is refilled percutaneously with strict asepsis. Programmable pumps are more expensive and need to be replaced when the battery fails, usually after 7–10 years. To support the provision of ITDD all the health care professionals involved, whether in primary or secondary care, must be trained in the techniques appropriate for managing patents with ITDD.

15.2 **Intrathecal drugs**

Many drugs have been given intrathecally, often almost empirically. Large-scale, long-term RCTs are needed to allow recommendations to be made about benefits and risks of ITDD in patients with neuropathic pain. Drug selection needs to be refined and validated. Data about neurotoxicity of spinal drugs is important. Preservative-free formulations should be used; drug stability in delivery systems and spinal fluid should be considered. Combining drugs with different mechanisms of action can produce synergy that may reduce side-effects.

15.2.1 **Opioids**

Most clinical experience with intrathecal therapy is with opioids; the efficacy of morphine in treating cancer and non-cancer pain is well established. Hydromorphone is a faster acting, more potent opioid than morphine due to its greater lipophilicity; it probably has fewer side effects as it has a smaller supra-spinal distribution. Diamorphine is only available for use in the United Kingdom and there is much less evidence about its efficacy and safety than other opioids. It cannot be used in fully implantable devices because there have been reports of pumps stalling due to corrosion of internal components when they have been filled with high concentrations of diamorphine. Opioids should be first-line therapy in most cases; ziconotide can also now be considered first-line; low IT doses should be used initially whilst reducing systemic opioid administration and gradually titrating the IT dose as needed. Patients with neuropathic pain may require higher IT doses than patients with nociceptive pain, especially with monotherapy. Central side-effects are often greater with hydrophilic drugs than with lipophilic drugs. Other opioid-induced adverse effects include emesis, itch, peripheral oedema, arthralgia, urinary retention, and endocrine or immune complications. Switching IT opioids can sometimes restore efficacy and reduce side-effects.

15.2.2 **Local anaesthetics**

Local anaesthetics given with opioids may reduce opioid tolerance. Bupivacaine is commonly used; ropivacaine and levobupivacaine are less cardiotoxic, but there is little evidence that they are better than bupivacaine for IT use. Several studies have demonstrated the effectiveness of addition of bupivacaine in those patients whom treatment with intrathecal morphine was inadequate. Side effects, e.g. leg weakness are fairly common with high doses e.g. more than 15mg/day (unlicensed use); urinary retention and orthostatic hypotension are less common

15.2.3 **Clonidine**

Clonidine has a synergistic effect with opioids (see Chapter 18) and can be a useful adjunct to spinal opioids for those patients with neuropathic pain. IT clonidine may cause sedation, fatigue, dry mouth, impaired bowel function, bradycardia, and hypotension (the latter especially with abrupt cessation). Animal models and case reports suggest that IT clonidine (<50 µg daily) may enhance analgesia from spinal cord stimulation (SCS) in some neuropathic pain states amd there is evidence for clinical efficacy in treating neuropathic from a number of studies.

15.2.4 **Baclofen**

Baclofen is a gamma amino butyric acid-B ($GABA_B$) agonist that has been used clinically by the IT route since the late 1980s for the treatment of children with cerebral palsy or adults with spasticity due to spinal cord injury or multiple sclerosis that does not respond to oral therapy. Low starting doses and slow titration are needed. Patients with implanted systems for the delivery of high dose baclofen are at risk if there is malfunction of the pump and/or spinal catheter system leading to sudden cessation of IT baclofen delivery; this may case severe neurological consequences or even death. Dyspnoea associated with increased muscle tone may be an important indicator of baclofen withdrawal. While increased spasticity is usually caused by drug tolerance or other factors, pruritis appears to be a good clinical indicator of baclofen withdrawal; this is clinically relevant when considering if a change in symptoms are a result of drug tolerance or a drug delivery problem. Other common side effects include sedation and muscle weakness.

15.2.5 **Ziconotide**

Ziconotide is a non-opioid analgesic that has been developed as a treatment for patients with severe chronic pain. It is derived from the venom of the marine snail Conus magus. It is a highly selective, potent, and reversible blocker of neuronal N-type voltage-sensitive calcium channels, with analgesic efficacy. It can be delivered only as an IT continuous infusion. It must be titrated very slowly over a number of weeks to minimize the adverse effects that were common in early studies due to fast titration and high dosing. Adverse effects at higher doses include dizziness, blurred vision, nystagmus, sedation, and psychomimetic effects. There is little tolerance after prolonged use. Ziconotide has a favourable risk/benefit ratio with advantages over several currently available IT therapies for pain. It is the only currently available drug for intrathecal use to have undergone randomized, placebo-controlled trials. Based on these and on increasing experience a panel of experts have recommended that ziconotide is considered as a first line choice of drug with morphine and hydromorphone. It appears to work more efficiently for neuropathic pain states but has also been used for patients with nociceptive pain and mixed pain. Adverse side effects reported in trials include elevated creatine kinase, sedation, somnolence, nausea, headache, neuropsychiatric symptoms (e.g. depression, confusion and cognitive impairment), ataxia, and abnormal gait.

15.2.6 Ketamine

Ketamine is a non-competitive N-methyl d-aspartate (NMDA) receptor antagonist that alters pain perception at spinal level. Concerns about toxicity after neuraxial use of racemic ketamine have led to the IT use of the preservative-free active compound, S(+)-ketamine (see Chapter 13). The S(+) active enantiomer has been considered less neurotoxic than the racemic mixture of ketamine. Clinical data suggest that ketamine may be advantageous in treating postoperative and severe intractable pain syndromes that are not alleviated by increasing IT opioid escalation. There are cases of severe neuropathic cancer pain that have been treated successfully by IT infusion of morphine, bupivacaine, clonidine, and S(+)-ketamine. In summary IT S(+)-ketamine can only be recommended as a last resort therapy due to the lack of preclinical safety data and conflicting information about its efficacy.

15.2.7 Other drugs

There are a number of other drugs that have undergone limited trials to assess their safety and efficacy for use IT.

Midazolam is a benzodiazepine receptor agonist. It has been shown in animals to potentiate the antinociceptive effect of opioids in the spinal cord. There are a number of case reports of improvements in severe cancer pain with the addition of IT midazolam to opioid and or local anaesthetics.

Gabapentin administered by intrathecal bolus in rodent models reduced mechanical allodynia and thermal hyperalgesia associated with central sensitization, tissue injury, inflammation and nerve injury. It has no effect on acute nociception. It has not undergone human trials.

Spinal prostaglandin synthesis may play a role in acute pain and the generation or maintenance of central sensitization. Animal studies have shown that IT ketorolac induces a potent analgesic effect. A phase 1 study in humans found no adverse effects with the use of IT ketorolac although it did not reduce pain due to a heat stimulus.

Animal models also provide insights into future IT therapies. Melatonin agonists can reduce the generation, development, and maintenance of central sensitization in neuropathic pain models. Nerve growth factor reverses neuropathic pain symptoms and restores opioid efficacy in animal models of neuropathic pain.

15.2.8 Algorithm for the selection of intrathecal drugs

The 2007 Polyanalgesic Consensus Conference on intrathecal drug delivery developed an algorithm (Figure 15.2) that reflects the current best available evidence and arranges drugs in a hierarchy according to safety, efficacy and broad clinical experience.

15.3 Neurolytic blocks

15.3.1 Background

Neurolysis in the peripheral nervous system has been replaced by other strategies as it is unlikely to produce long-lasting analgesia and may lead to deafferentation pain. However neurolytic blocks are useful in some patients with trigeminal neuralgia, cancer, or ischaemic vascular conditions, when pain is often fully or partly neuropathic. Neurolytic sympathetic plexus blocks (NSPB) can relieve pain and improve quality of life in cancer patients. A study of 60 patients with abdominal or pelvic cancer pain (in 2 different disease phases) compared NSPB with pharmacological therapy alone, over eight weeks. Those who had NSPB early and later in their disease had a significant reduction of pain and opioid consumption, and a better quality of life than those who were pharmacologically managed. Opioid-related adverse effects were significantly greater in the drug-treated group. Occasional complications were transitory. NSPB for the management of cancer pain should be considered earlier in the disease, and calls into question the World Health Organization recommendations of using blocks as a last resort. Patients must be carefully assessed and investigated to determine whether or not a nerve block is feasible and likely to help. The procedure and its benefits and burdens must be explained to the patient. Radiological imaging, with or without contrast, is helpful for some blocks and mandatory for others, e.g. coeliac plexus block. A temporary local anaesthetic block may predict the response to a neurolytic block. The use of nerve blocks as prognostic tools can be difficult because of confounding factors, e.g. systemic absorption of local anaesthetics leading to analgesia and placebo response.

Figure 15.2 Recommendations for the management of Pain by Intrathecal Drug Delivery (reproduced with permission from the Polyanalgesic Consensus Conference 2007)

15.3.2 **Trigeminal blocks**

Microvascular decompression via posterior fossa surgery, percutaneous gasserian glycerol neurolysis, balloon compression, and radiofrequency trigeminal lesion can all be used to treat trigeminal neuralgia that is resistant to medical therapy. These ganglion-level interventions are more effective than peripheral procedures, but no approach can be totally relied on to produce long term analgesia. All techniques are neuro-destructive and can cause sensory loss and dysaesthesia. At longer follow-up intervals, microvascular decompression is predicted to be the most cost-effective procedure, and should be considered as the preferred operation for patients if their risk for general anaesthesia is acceptable. Percutaneous surgery may be better for older patients with medically unresponsive trigeminal neuralgia.

15.3.3 **Lumbar sympathectomy**

Interruption of the lumbar sympathetic chain can provide pain relief for some patients with vascular neuropathic pain, e.g. those with non-reconstructable critical limb ischaemia. Pre-operative ankle-brachial index has prognostic value, with clinical improvement if it is >0.3. Diabetes, angiography, palpable popliteal pulses, age, and sex are not predictive of success; results are not as good in smokers. Patients with rest pain alone do better than those with gangrene, especially of the big toe. Once gangrene is more extensive, then sympathectomy is probably not helpful for limb salvage, but may help neuropathic pain and stump healing. When considering non-vascular neuropathic pain e.g. CRPS, the use of sympathectomy in clinical practice is based on very weak evidence (see Chapter 8). Some animal data has suggested that sympathectomy is effective when the animals show severe mechanical hypersensitivity, but more detailed clinical research is needed. Complications include postural hypotension (especially if bilateral block is performed), genito-femoral neuritis, sexual dysfunction, renal damage, lumbar plexus damage, injection into the aortic wall leading to dissection, and intraperitoneal, epidural, or intrathecal injection.

15.3.4 **Coeliac plexus block (CPB) and superior hypogastric plexus block (SHPB)**

Coeliac plexus block (CPB) can provide good pain relief in some visceral pains that may be associated with visceral hyperalgesia, and thus be considered as partly neuropathic. CPB is used for patients with pain from upper abdominal cancer, and superior hypogastric plexus block (SHPB) for cancer pain arising from the pelvis and perineum. The role of neurolytic sympathetic blocks in advanced cancer, when pain syndromes may involve other structures, e.g. posterior abdominal and pelvic walls, is less clear. There are several different approaches to CPB, including retro-crural, transcrural, transaortic, anterior, and greater splanchnic nerve block; complications can occur (Box 15.2). In a survey of 36 patients with advanced pancreatic or pelvic cancer pain, a neuropathic component was more common in those with pelvic cancers; these patients had less pain relief after neurolytic blocks than patients with pain due to pancreatic cancer.

15.3.5 Intrathecal neurolytic injection of sacrococcygeal nerve roots

Intrathecal neurolysis was commonly used for unilateral pain in the thoracic and lumbar area. Serious adverse effects such as motor blockade are possible, and now with the advent of spinal drug delivery, this technique is not used commonly. However, it still has value in the management of some cancer pain problems, e.g. pelvic and perineal pain.

Box 15.2 Complications of coeliac plexus block

- Local pain
- Diarrhoea
  - Usually resolves within 48 hours (if not consider octreotide)
- Hypotension
  - Usually resolves within 48 hours
  - Use adequate hydration and support stockings
  - Vasopressors occasionally needed
- Neurological complications
  - Lower extremity weakness and paraesthesiae
  - Lumbar plexus damage
  - Epidural placement of neurolytic agent
  - Lumbar puncture
  - Urinary or faecal incontinence
  - Sexual dysfunction
  - Paraplegia
- Significant non-neurological adverse effects
  - Pneumothorax
  - Shoulder, chest, and pleuritic pain
  - Hiccup
  - Haematuria
  - Aortic dissection
  - Silent gastric perforation

15.4 **Intracerebroventricular drug delivery (ICVDD)**

Drugs can be delivered directly into the cerebral ventricles; this requires a surgical transcranial approach, with its accompanying morbidity. Intracerebroventricular drug delivery (ICVDD) can be useful for those with neuropathic head pain, usually due to cancer. Uncontrolled studies suggest that ICVDD is at least as effective as other neuraxial treatments, and may be successful for patients whose pain is resistant to other therapies.

Key references

Abram, S.E. (2000). Neural blockade for neuropathic pain. *Clin J Pain*, **16**, S56–61.

Ballantyne, J.C., Carwood, C.M. (2005). Comparative efficacy of epidural, subarachnoid, and intra-cerebroventricular opioids in patients with pain due to cancer. Cochrane Database of Systematic Reviews, Issue 1; CD005178.

Deer T., Krames E.S., Hassenbusch S.J. Polyanalgesic Consensus Conference (2007): Recommendations for the management of Pain by Intrathecal Drug Delivery: Neuromodulation 4:300-328.

Hassenbusch S.J.,Portenoy R.K., Cousins M., *et al.* Polyanalgesic Consensus Conference 2003: An Update on the management of Pain by Intraspinal delivery-Report of an Expert Panel. *J Pain Symptom Man*, (2004) **6**, 540–63.

Hicks, F. and Simpson, K.H. (2004). *Nerve blocks in palliative care.* Oxford University Press, Oxford.

Mailis, A., Furlan, A. (2003). Sympathectomy for neuropathic pain. Cochrane Database of Systematic Reviews, Issue 2; CD002918.

Prager, J.P. (2002). Neuraxial medication delivery: the development and maturity of a concept for treating chronic pain of spinal origin. *Spine*, **27**, 2593–605.

Turner, J.A., Sears J.M., Loeser J.D. (2007). Programmable Intrathecal Opioid Delivery systems for Chronic Non-cancer Pain: A Systematic Reviewof Effectivenss and Complications. *Clin J Pain*, **2**, 180–95.

Chapter 16

Transcutaneous electrical nerve stimulation (TENS) and acupuncture

Mark I. Johnson

Key points

- TENS and acupuncture are simple and generally safe methods of stimulating peripheral nerves and muscles close to the site of pain in order to modulate nociceptive input to the spinal cord
- TENS can be useful for peripheral neuropathic pain and analgesic effects are often felt immediately
- Best results occur when patients are given a supervised trial of TENS to guide electrode placement and stimulation settings, although TENS is widely available to the public
- Pain relief from acupuncture is generally delayed following treatment but often outlasts the stimulation period (in contrast to TENS)
- There is a dearth of good-quality evidence to guide decisions regarding TENS and acupuncture in neuropathic pain. However, both have few adverse effects, can be combined easily with drug therapy, and are always worth a trial in a patient who has not responded to other treatments.

16.1 Transcutaneous electrical nerve stimulation (TENS)

16.1.1 Background

Transcutaneous electrical nerve stimulation (TENS) is the delivery of pulsed electrical currents across the intact surface of the skin to stimulate the underlying nerves. A battery-powered, portable

Figure 16.1 Standard TENS device

Self-adhesive electrodes

Electrode leads

Portable current
generator

stimulating device is used to generate the currents, and conducting
pads called electrodes are used to deliver the currents through the
skin (Figure 16.1).

TENS is non-invasive, easy to administer, and has few side-effects
or drug interactions. TENS effects are immediate for most patients
and there is no potential for toxicity or overdose. TENS treatment is
inexpensive when compared to long-term drug therapy. At the time
of writing, a standard TENS device costs approximately £30 (approx.
€43) and running costs (batteries and electrodes) are low. Patients
can administer TENS themselves at home and titrate the dosage of
treatment as required. Patients can purchase TENS devices over the
counter without medical prescription, although new patients should
always be given a supervised trial of TENS from a practitioner experienced in the principles of application. Patients should be provided
with a point of contact to troubleshoot any problems with TENS.

16.1.2 **Biological rationale and plausibility**

The physiological purpose of TENS is to selectively activate large-
diameter non-noxious afferents (A) without activating smaller-
diameter nociceptive afferents (Aδ and C). Physiological studies have
shown that afferent input inhibits ongoing activity in second-order
nociceptive neurons in the dorsal horn of the spinal cord.

16.1.3 **Clinical effectiveness**

Clinical experience suggests that TENS is useful for neuropathic pain, irrespective of cause and whether or not there is a sympathetic component. TENS appears to be more effective for neuropathic pains of peripheral rather than central origin, especially if there is a loss of large-fibre input. However, there are few good-quality randomized controlled clinical trials.

A European Federation of Neurological Societies (EFNS) Task Force evaluated nine controlled trials (200 patients) on TENS for neuropathic pain and concluded that TENS was better than placebo (level C evidence). A Cochrane review on TENS for chronic pain in 2008 included 25 RCTs (1,281 participants) of which only one RCT was specifically on neuropathic pain. Evidence was inconclusive. A Cochrane review on electrical stimulation for post-stroke pain was also inconclusive.

Published trials suggest that TENS is beneficial for peripheral neuropathic pain due to post-herpetic neuralgia, trigeminal neuralgia, phantom limb and stump pain, radiculopathies (cervical, thoracic, and lumbar), diabetes, and entrapment neuropathies such as carpal tunnel syndrome. TENS has been used for neuropathic cancer pain caused by nerve compression by a neoplasm or infiltration by a tumor, and for iatrogenic neuralgias such as post-mastectomy and post-thoracotomy pains. TENS may also be useful for complex regional pain syndromes type I (reflex sympathetic dystrophy) and type II (causalgia), and central pain states following stroke and post-traumatic spinal cord injury pain.

16.2 **TENS: principles of use**

16.2.1 **Electrode position**

TENS electrodes must be positioned on healthy skin where sensation is intact, so it is important to check skin sensation prior to application. TENS may aggravate neuropathic pain, especially when there is mechanical (tactile) allodynia. Therefore, electrodes should be positioned along the main nerves well proximal to the site of pain in the first instance. Alternatively, electrodes can be positioned on a contralateral dermatome or paravertebrally at the appropriate spinal segment. For most other types of pain, TENS electrodes are placed around the site of pain so that paraesthesia can be directed into the painful area (Figure 16.2a and b).

16.2.2 **Electrical characteristics of TENS**

The potential number of TENS protocols is vast (Figure 13.3). Theoretically, selective activation of large-diameter afferents occurs best

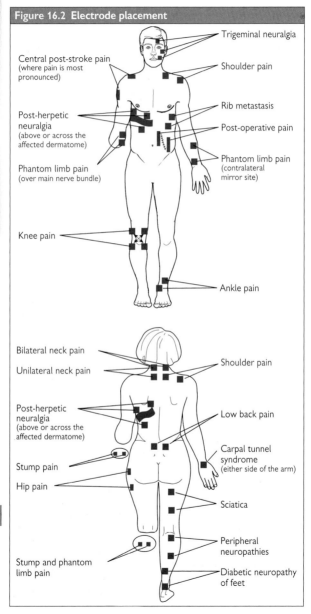

Figure 16.2 Electrode placement

Trigeminal neuralgia

Shoulder pain

Central post-stroke pain (where pain is most pronounced)

Rib metastasis

Post-operative pain

Post-herpetic neuralgia (above or across the affected dermatome)

Phantom limb pain (contralateral mirror site)

Phantom limb pain (over main nerve bundle)

Knee pain

Ankle pain

Bilateral neck pain

Shoulder pain

Unilateral neck pain

Post-herpetic neuralgia (above or across the affected dermatome)

Low back pain

Carpal tunnel syndrome (either side of the arm)

Stump pain

Hip pain

Sciatica

Peripheral neuropathies

Stump and phantom limb pain

Diabetic neuropathy of feet

Figure 16.3 Output characteristics

High | Low | Channel 1 | Channel 2

Pulse intensity

Pulse intensity 0...60mA | Pulse intensity 0...60mA | Continuous pattern (C)

Burst pattern (B)

B C M
Pulse pattern
50∞<2 50∞<s | 1Hz 200Hz
Pulse duration | Pulse frequency

Modulated pattern (M)

Short | Long | High | Low

Pulse duration | Battery | Pulse frequency

with high-frequency (e.g. 10–200 pulses per second), low-intensity currents with pulse durations between 50–500μs. In practice, activation of large-diameter afferents is recognized by 'strong but comfortable' paraesthesiae beneath the electrodes and patients are instructed to titrate the intensity of currents to achieve this effect. Patients are encouraged to experiment with TENS settings for pulse frequency, pulse pattern, and pulse duration because optimal settings remain unknown.

16.2.3 Timing and dosage
TENS effects are often immediate and are maximal when the device is switched on. Hence, patients should keep the device switched on whenever they need pain relief. Patients can leave electrodes *in situ* and administer TENS intermittently throughout the day, providing they attend to skin care underneath the electrodes as minor skin irritation may occur. Patients should wash skin after TENS and should apply electrodes to adjacent fresh skin on a regular basis.

16.2.4 Contraindications and precautions
Patients with cardiac pacemakers or with cardiac problems should not use TENS, unless the situation has been discussed with their cardiologist. TENS should not be administered over the abdomen or pelvis during pregnancy because its effects on fetal development are unknown and currents could inadvertently cause uterine contractions. Practitioners should be cautious when giving TENS to patients with epilepsy as it may be difficult to exclude it as a potential cause of a seizure. TENS should not be given to patients with a history of autonomic reactions to tactile allodynia such as syncope, or to patients

with compromised circulation such as thrombosis. Decisions are left to the discretion of the medical practitioner.

TENS should not be applied internally (mouth), over areas of broken or damaged skin, or over the anterior part of the neck as this may cause an acute hypotensive response. TENS should not be used while operating motor vehicles or potentially hazardous equipment or while in the shower or bath. It can be used at bedtime providing the device has a timer so that it automatically switches off. It can also be used on children providing they understand what to expect during the process.

16.2.5 Acupuncture-like TENS (AL-TENS)

This technique is a form of hyperstimulation and can be used when patients do not respond to conventional TENS. Electrodes are placed over pain-related dermatomes, myotomes, acupuncture points and trigger points. Non-painful muscle twitching is often produced during stimulation using intermittent bursts of pulses generated by the TENS device (Figure 16.3). The resultant input from small-diameter muscle afferents activates descending inhibitory pain pathways which produces pain relief that outlasts the stimulation period. AL-TENS is given intermittently throughout the day, e.g. 20 minutes, three times a day.

Clinical experience suggests that AL-TENS is useful for radiating neuropathic pain such as sciatica and cervical rhizopathy. A dual-channel device (four electrodes) can be used to deliver conventional TENS over the nerve root as it emerges from the spinal cord and AL-TENS over the main muscle mass of the radiating pain. AL-TENS can be applied to contralateral myotomes when it is not possible to achieve TENS paraesthesia at the site of pain due to hyperaesthesia, hypoaesthesia, or dysaesthesia.

A variety of TENS-like devices are available on the market but their use is limited because of a lack of research evidence. They include microcurrent stimulation, transcutaneous spinal electroanalgesia (TSE), interferential therapy (IFT), and Pain® Gone pens.

16.3 Acupuncture

16.3.1 Background

Acupuncture is the technique of inserting fine needles through the skin into selected points in the body to stimulate underlying nerve and muscle tissue. Additional stimulation is achieved by 'twirling' the inserted needle or by passing mild currents through pairs of needles using a portable electrical stimulator, termed 'electroacupuncture'.

Originally, acupuncture was based on the principles of traditional Chinese medicine where it was believed that acupuncture could alter the flow of vital energies of life (Yin and Yang) along energy channels or meridians. Nowadays, many medical practitioners adopt a Western approach to acupuncture which involves diagnosis according to orthodox medicine.

16.3.2 Biological rationale and plausibility

There is no convincing evidence for the existence of meridians as finite structures. Evidence that acupuncture points correspond to anatomical structures such as nerve bundles, nerves emerging from deep to superficial motor points, myofascial trigger points, and perivascular plexi has been challenged.

Needling during acupuncture stimulates high-threshold receptors and/or their afferents (Aδ and C), leading to segmental and extrasegmental modulation of nociceptive input. Post-stimulation effects have been attributed to activity in descending inhibitory pain pathways, the release of endogenous opioids, and positive-feedback neural circuitry in the mesolimbic region of the brain. Studies using rat models of neuropathic pain suggest that electroacupuncture can reduce mechanical allodynia. Acupuncture affects activity in the autonomic nervous system and may improve microcirculation through axon reflexes and the release of vasoactive substances such as calcitonin gene-related peptide and substance P.

16.3.3 Clinical effectiveness

Clinical experience suggests that acupuncture is beneficial for nociceptive and musculoskeletal pain but is less effective for neuropathic pain. Beneficial effects have been reported on phantom limb pain, diabetic neuropathy, and neurogenic pruritus. A randomized, placebo-controlled, multicentre clinical trial found that acupuncture was no more effective than placebo for peripheral neuropathy in human immunodeficiency virus (HIV) infected individuals. A recent systematic review concluded that rigorous clinical trials do not support acupuncture as an effective analgesic adjunctive method for pain related to cancer, including neuropathic pain. However, there are insufficient good-quality randomized controlled trials to guide clinical decisions for neuropathic pain conditions. For this reason, acupuncture may be worth a trial in a patient who has not responded to other treatments or who cannot tolerate drug therapy. Acupuncture has few adverse effects and can be combined with drug therapy or TENS.

16.4 Acupuncture: principles of use

Formal training is required to administer acupuncture (www.medical-acupuncture.co.uk). The debate about what constitutes appropriate technique and adequate dose of acupuncture treatment is longstanding. Acupuncture treatment has many components and is much more than just needling, although by definition 'needle puncture' gives acupuncture its identity. The components of acupuncture needling procedures, and more recently 'dose', have been described (see STRICTA guidelines).

16.4.1 **Point selection**

The exact site and depth of penetration is determined by the practitioner and believed to be critical to outcome. Western practitioners choose points in accordance with known physiological and anatomical principles, e.g. dermatome, myotome, and sclerotome. The general consensus is to use points from innervated regions with properly functioning nerves. Direct stimulation of hyperaesthetic areas is avoided.

Needles should be placed proximal to the site of nerve damage or above a complete transection in spinal cord injuries. Needles could be placed to surround a stump scar for phantom limb pain or on trigger areas in the stump, providing they are not hyperaesthetic. In conditions like post-herpetic neuralgia or trigeminal neuralgia, practitioners would stimulate above and below the affected segment or use contralateral 'mirror' points.

Points are avoided in areas of skin where the nerve supply or circulation has been compromised, as in peripheral neuropathy. Stronger stimulation acupuncture techniques such as electroacupuncture are often used if distant points are chosen. Trigger points are often used for pains of musculoskeletal origin. In practice, optimal point selection is achieved through a careful process of trial and error.

16.4.2 **Timing and dosage**

Acupuncturists typically use fine (0.2–0.3mm) disposable steel needles which are 30mm long. Needles are left in place for up to 30 minutes and may be intermittently manipulated to facilitate stimulation. Patients may report sensations of heaviness, soreness, a local dull ache, referred pain, numbness, and/or paraesthesia during acupuncture.

In general, pain relief from acupuncture outlasts the period of stimulation and may persist for several days or weeks. The onset of analgesia may be delayed and some patients experience an initial transient increase in pain in the first 48 hours. A typical course of acupuncture consists of six to 12 treatments given once per week. Pain relief may be cumulative over time. Patients may attend acupuncture clinics for 'top-up' sessions thereafter.

16.4.3 **Contraindications and precautions**

Acupuncture is relatively safe when administered by a trained practitioner. Contraindications include bleeding disorders, anticoagulant medication, placing needles close to a pregnant uterus, and patients with a needle phobia.

Electroacupuncture is contraindicated for patients with cardiac pacemakers. Serious adverse events such as pneumothorax, cardiac tamponade, and fatalities due to needle infection are rare, although minor events such as pain due to the needles, tiredness, and bleeding are much more common. Occasionally patients may feel faint.

Key references

Barlas, P., Lundeberg, T. (2006). Transcutaneous electrical nerve stimulation and acupuncture. In: S.B. McMahaon and M. Koltzenburg (ed.) *Melzack and Wall's textbook of pain*, pp. 583–90. Elsevier Churchill Livingstone, Philadelphia.

Cruccu G., Aziz T.Z., Garcia-Larrea L., Hansson P., Jensen T.S., Lefaucheur J.-P., Simpson B.A., Taylor R.S. (2007) EFNS guidelines on neurostimulation therapy for neuropathic pain. *European Journal of Neurology*, **14**, 952–70.

Johnson, M.I. (2008). Transcutaneous electrical nerve stimulation. In: T. Watson (ed.) *Electrotherapy: evidence-based practice*, pp. 253–296, Churchill Livingstone, Edinburgh, UK.

Lee, H., Schmidt, K., and Ernst, E. (2005). Acupuncture for the relief of cancer-related pain: a systematic review. *Eur. J. Pain*, **9**: 437–44.

MacPherson H., White A., Cummings M., Jobst K., Rose K., Niemtzow R. (2002); STandards for Reporting Interventions in Controlled Trails of Acupuncture. Standards for reporting interventions in controlled trials of acupuncture: The STRICTA recommendations. STandards for Reporting Interventions in Controlled Trails of Acupuncture. *Acupunct Med*, **20**(1), 22–5.

National Health Service Centre for Reviews and Dissemination (2001). Acupuncture. *Effective Health Care Bulletin*, **7**, 1–2.

Nnoaham K.E., Kumbang J. (2008). Transcutaneous electrical nerve stimulation (TENS) for chronic pain. Cochrane Database of Systematic Reviews, Issue 2: CD003222.

Price, C.I., Pandyan, A.D. (2001). Electrical stimulation for preventing and treating post-stroke shoulder pain: a systematic Cochrane review. *Clin Rehab*, **15**, 5–19.

Shlay, J.C., Chaloner, K., Max, M.B., Flaws, B., Reichelderfer, P., Wentworth, D., *et al.* (1998). Acupuncture and amitriptyline for pain due to HIV-related peripheral neuropathy: a randomized controlled trial. *JAMA*, **280**, 1590–5.

White A., Cummings M., Barlas P., Cardini F., Filshie J., Foster N.E., Lundeberg T., Stener-Victorin E., Witt C. (2008). Defining an adequate dose of acupuncture using a neurophysiological approach — a narrative review of the literature. *Acupunct Med*, **26**(2), 111–20.

Chapter 17

Spinal cord stimulation

Brian A. Simpson

Key points

- Electricity has been used for centuries to relieve pain but spinal cord stimulation (SCS) came about with the Gate Control Theory in the 1960s
- SCS was originally thought simply to 'close the gate' by activating Aβ fibres but its effect is more complex. It is likely that it helps to normalize the dysfunction that manifests as neuropathic pain
- SCS is most effective for neuropathic and ischaemic pain, and is ineffective in nociceptive pain
- Electrodes are placed in the epidural space either via percutaneous needle or at open operation. The power source is usually implanted and is similar to a cardiac pacemaker
- SCS can produce significant benefits in terms of pain and function in up to 70% of patients with neuropathic pain, though more controlled trials are needed to establish long-term benefits.

17.1 Introduction

17.1.1 Electricity and pain relief

There is nothing new about the use of electricity to relieve pain. Natural sources, particularly electric fish and also the static electricity from amber, etc., were widely used for thousands of years. Man-made electricity dates from 1672 (electrostatic generator) and could be stored after 1745 (Leyden jar). Electroacupuncture is nearly 200 years old (1823) and peripheral nerve stimulation was also developed during the nineteenth century. It was very widely employed but its widespread misuse led to its ban in the USA in 1910. History nearly repeated itself in the 1970s and early 1980s with spinal cord stimulation (SCS).

17.1.2 **Modern neurostimulation**

The modern era of therapeutic neurostimulation was triggered in the 1960s by the gate theory of pain. It was the underlying principle, combined with a new appreciation of the plasticity of the nervous system and its tendency to generate pain when damaged, that fostered this modulatory approach along with a slow rejection of neurodestructive procedures. However, the combination of unreliable equipment, a lack of appreciation of the indications, and large numbers of practitioners each performing small numbers of procedures with inadequate follow-up almost led to its demise. Through improvements in each of these areas therapeutic neurostimulation not only survived but is developing rapidly, with many thousands of devices, mainly spinal cord stimulators, implanted annually worldwide. Despite the maturity and the breadth of the field, there are still fundamental issues to be resolved.

17.2 **Mechanism of action**

17.2.1 **Analgesic effects**

A great deal is still not known about how SCS works. The posterior columns have a key role and SCS is still sometimes referred to as 'dorsal column stimulation'. The large, myelinated, low-threshold Aβ afferent fibres, whose activity was proposed to 'close the gate' by inhibiting simultaneous nociceptive activity in small, unmyelinated C fibres, have collateral branches which ascend in the posterior columns. The rationale of SCS originally was to activate these Aβ collaterals, which transmit signals from mechanoreceptors: the electrophysiological equivalent of 'rubbing it better'.

There is an essential topographic element in that the electrodes must not only be ipsilateral (for unilateral pain), but stimulation must also evoke paraesthesiae which cover the painful area. Although the debate about the relative contributions of a supraspinal long-loop mechanism and an action at segmental level in the spinal cord continues, it is obvious that SCS does not simply close the gate on nociceptive input; it is not effective against nociceptive pain.

In animal models of neuropathic pain, the suppression of allodynia and of neuronal hyperexcitability in the dorsal horn of the spinal cord by SCS has been linked to an increased release of gamma amino butyric acid (GABA) and a decreased release of excitatory amino acids. Adenosine is also involved and neuronal activity changes have been demonstrated in brainstem nuclei.

17.2.2 **Anti-ischaemic effect**

SCS has an anti-ischaemic effect and the extent to which this underlies the analgesic effect in ischaemic pain is not yet established. It also stabilizes the vasomotor and sudomotor abnormalities in complex regional pain syndrome (CRPS) to a variable extent and appears to be able to reduce gastrointestinal spasm. There is as yet no consensus as to whether the autonomic effects represent modulation of ongoing sympathetic efferent activity or an antidromic activation of primary afferents.

Neuropathic pain is the product of a complex dysfunction of the nervous system and it seems that SCS produces a degree of normalization, probably by several mechanisms whose relative contribution varies in different conditions.

17.3 **Selection of cases**

17.3.1 Indications

The main indications for SCS are now well established and comprise essentially neuropathic and ischaemic pain. SCS does not influence nociceptive (e.g. arthritic and acute post-operative) pain. Some neuropathic syndromes respond better than others (Box 17.1). It should be remembered that SCS is not the only form of neurostimulation available; cases that do not respond adequately might respond to peripheral nerve, sacral root, or brain stimulation.

Box 17.1 Indications for spinal cord stimulation

Good indications
- Complex regional pain syndrome
- Neuropathic limb pain following spinal surgery ('failed back or neck surgery syndrome')
- Peripheral nerve damage
- Brachial plexus damage (not avulsion)
- Angina pectoris
- Peripheral vascular disease (obstructive and vasospastic).

Intermediate indications
- Amputation pain (stump pain better than phantom pain)
- Axial pain following spinal surgery
- Intercostal neuralgia (incl. post-thoracotomy pain)
- Spinal cord (partial) damage
- Diabetic neuropathy.

Poor indications
- Supraspinal central pain
- Perineal and anorectal pain.

Not indicated
- Complete spinal cord transection
- Nerve root avulsion
- Non-ischaemic nociceptive pain.

Although it has long been known that SCS can stabilize the hyperexcitable neurogenic bladder, the exciting prospect has only very recently emerged that visceral pain, such as in severe irritable bowel syndrome and oesophageal spasm, and pancreatic and chronic post-laparotomy pain, may also respond to SCS. The neuropathic element of these conditions and others, e.g. interstitial cystitis, is now increasingly recognized; autonomic dysfunction is of course a feature of several of the more established indications of SCS.

17.3.2 Other considerations

There are very few contraindications (Box 17.2). Case selection is crucially important and the diagnosis alone is insufficient; it is not understood why patients with the same favourable diagnosis (see Box 17.1) may respond differently. Trial stimulation via temporary external connections is not a complete solution. Even when conducted thoroughly over a month or more, the resulting long-term success rate in neuropathic pain rarely exceeds 65–70%. The 1-in-3 failure rate reflects both the clinical complexity of many patients with neuropathic pain and the methodology of trial stimulation (see Assessment of outcome, p.167). Trials do not effectively exclude placebo responders and desperate wishful thinkers, but may exclude others who would obtain a useful effect in the long term but who do not attain the arbitrary pass mark.

Appraisal by a psychologist has not been shown to improve the success rate overall, but it does provide an important opportunity for detailed assessment and counselling.Patients' expectations must be appropriate: complete abolition of the pain should not be expected, although it can occur; in mixed syndromes any nociceptive element will not respond; a favourable modification of the pain should permit a reduction or cessation of medication and improved activity with concomitant increase in the ability to cope with any residual pain. SCS will not by itself, however, convert a miserable life into a rewarding one.

Box 17.2 Contraindications to spinal cord stimulation

Absolute
- Demand-type cardiac pacemaker
- Implanted cardiac defibrillator
- Uncontrolled coagulopathy
- Sepsis.

Relative
- Cognitive impairment.

17.4 **Equipment and methodology**

17.4.1 **Electrode placement**

The electrodes are placed in the posterior epidural space by one of two methods. 'Wire' or 'catheter' systems can be inserted percutaneously via a Tuohy needle, usually under local anaesthesia. This is minimally invasive, allows feedback to optimize the positioning, and the implanter does not have to be a surgeon. On the negative side these systems usually cannot penetrate epidural scarring (but can penetrate the dura), are electrically inefficient, and are more prone to dislodgement than are the alternative plate electrodes. The latter require an open operation and are often referred to as 'surgical' electrodes or leads. They are more efficient and more secure and there is some evidence that they are more effective, but their insertion usually requires a general anaesthetic and entails a bigger procedure (Figure 17.1).

Both rostrocaudal and lateral positioning of the electrodes determine the distribution of the evoked paraesthesiae. Four available contacts were the norm for many years (Figure 17.2) but more complex modern systems (Figure 17.1) give more flexibility, particularly when combined with multichannel technology which allows electronic 'steering'.

Figure 17.1 Percutaneously implantable (left) and surgical (right) electrode systems for spinal cord stimulation. (Courtesy of Advanced Bionics, Inc.)

Figure 17.2 Radiograph showing four-contact plate electrode system (Lamitrode-22™; Reproduced courtesy of Advanced Neuromodulation Systems Inc.) in the lower thoracic spine

17.4.2 **Power sources**

The power source can be either an implanted pulse generator (IPG) similar to a cardiac pacemaker (Figure 17.3) or an external transmitter linked to an internal receiver-transducer by radiofrequency (RF) coupling from an antenna on the skin. The former is less cumbersome but the power source will become depleted after an average of about five or six years (newer devices may last longer) depending on usage; surgical replacement will then be required, which also represents a significant recurring cost. Rechargeable systems have recently become available and may obviate the need for RF systems. IPGs are programmed by telemetry to adjust frequency, pulse width and amplitude, selection of contacts and their polarity, plus various cycling options. The patient has a home programmer to select pre-set programmes and adjust the amplitude. RF transmitters can be similarly programmed.

The relatively high initial cost belies the increasingly well-established cost-effectiveness with break-even occurring by 3 years.

17.5 **Assessment of outcome**

17.5.1 **Assessment measures**

It might be assumed that assessing the effect of SCS in neuropathic pain would be straightforward. In some clearly successful cases it is, but in many others the clinical complexity, including the effects of long-term pain, long-term disability, and long-term medication, confuses the issue. The confusion is compounded by inappropriate reliance on numerical rating scales of pain intensity, by the difference between clinical and statistical significance, by the influence of memory, by the natural variability over time, and by the lack of a meaningful definition of success (50% reduction in pain is not meaningful in a long-term condition). Some of these flaws also affect trial stimulation (see above).

Box 17.3 **Complications and other adverse considerations**

Complications
- Infection (2–5%)
- Dural puncture (percutaneous leads)
- Epidural haematoma (rare)
- Permanent neurological damage (very rare)
- Lead migration (commoner with percutaneous than plate electrodes and in the cervical spine)
- Lead fracture
- Failure of other components.

Drawbacks/warnings
- Cannot generally undergo magnetic resonance imaging (MRI)
- Cannot receive therapeutic diathermy
- Special precautions with surgical diathermy
- Cannot drive with stimulator switched on
- Triggering security systems (carry an ID card or bracelet).

17.5.2 **Evidence of benefit**

For the treatment as a whole there is very little class I evidence. There are only three randomized controlled trials with appropriate follow-up periods, one for reflex sympathetic dystrophy, now known as CRPS type I, and two for failed back surgery syndrome. More are needed but the outcome measures used must be appropriate and holistic.

Unlike medication, SCS has virtually no side-effects. It does of course have risks, complications, and disadvantages (Box 17.3) and should be practised by experienced multidisciplinary teams. Difficulties aside, delivering significant benefit in up to 70% of appropriately selected patients for whom nothing else has been effective makes SCS a very useful treatment.

17.6 **The future**

- Devices will become more sophisticated but some of the requirements—versatility, reliability, small size, longevity, and low cost – may be mutually exclusive
- The conditions treated will be better understood, e.g. CRPS, thereby improving case selection
- Both case selection and outcome assessment will improve.
- New indications (e.g. visceral pain) will be established
- Earlier implementation may modify disease natural history, rather than simply palliating.
- More high-quality clinical and scientific research will be published.

Key references

Kemler, M.A., De Vet, H.C., Barendse, G.A., Van Den Wildenberg, F.A., Van Kleef, M. (2004). The effect of spinal cord stimulation in patients with chronic reflex sympathetic dystrophy: two years' follow-up of the randomized controlled trial. *Ann. Neurol*, **55**, 13–18.

Kumar, K., Taylor, R.S., Jaques, L., *et al.* (2007). Spinal cord stimulation versus conventional medical management for neuropathic pain: A multicentre randomised controlled trial in patients with failed back surgery syndrome. *Pain*, **132**, 179-88.

Melzack, R., Wall, P.D. (1965). Pain mechanisms: a new theory. *Science*, **150**, 971–9.

North, R.B., Kidd, D.H., Farrokhi, F., Piantadosi, S.A. (2005). Spinal cord stimulation versus repeated lumbosacral spine surgery for chronic pain: a randomized, controlled trial. *Neurosurgery*, **56**, 98–107.

Simpson, B.A., (ed.) (2003). *Electrical stimulation and the relief of pain* Elsevier, Amsterdam.

Simpson, K., Stannard, C. (ed.) (2005). *Spinal cord stimulation for the management of pain: recommendations for best clinical practice.* British Pain Society, London.

Chapter 18

Drug synergy and sequencing

Michael I. Bennett

Key points

- Combinations of drugs that work through different mechanisms can result in additive or synergistic effects that may improve control of pain, reduce side-effects, or both
- Most evidence comes from studies of co-analgesics with opioids and is derived from both animal and clinical research
- Although number needed to treat (NNT) is used to compare drug effectiveness, this method may miss some benefits, overestimate reliability (if confidence intervals are wide), and may detract from number needed to harm (NNH)
- Stepwise or parallel approaches to drug combinations have equal merit
- First-line approaches can be initiated in primary care but second- and third-line approaches will require increasingly close liaison with specialist pain management services.

18.1 Rationale for combination treatment

18.1.1 Drug synergy

In neuropathic pain, the main purpose of utilizing drug combinations is to improve pain control and reduce adverse effects. By combining drugs with different mechanisms of action, additive or even synergistic analgesic effects can be achieved whilst minimizing adverse effects. This results in better pain control and improved concordance with drug treatment.

Drug synergy is produced when the effects of a drug combination are greater than when the individual drug effects are simply added together. In other words, synergy is a situation where one plus one equals three. Demonstrating synergy in clinical practice can be difficult but as an example, if 1mg of drug A plus 1mg of drug B results in the same effect as 5mg of drug A or drug B alone, then synergy is taking place. If the combination results in the same effect as 2mg of A or B alone, then the effects are additive, not synergistic.

There are two broad types of drug synergy based on the nature of the interaction: pharmacodynamic or pharmacokinetic. Pharmacodynamic synergy results from two drugs with different actions directed at a similar target or physiological system. A good example of this is the use of rifampicin and isoniazid in the treatment of tuberculosis. Pharmacokinetic synergy results when one drug influences the absorption, distribution, biotransformation, or elimination of another drug. A classic example of this is the combination of amoxicillin with clavulanic acid; the latter prevents the breakdown of the former by beta-lactamase producing bacteria.

18.1.2 Evidence from pre-clinical studies

Animal studies have shown powerful evidence for short term (hours or days) drug synergy in neuropathic pain. In these studies, differences in mechanisms of action of individual analgesic drugs are exploited and their neurochemical and physiological effects can be studied in great detail. For example, sub-anti-nociceptive doses of intrathecal morphine (i.e. doses that do not prevent the sensation of pain) are enhanced when combined with oral gabapentin. This anti-nociceptive effect is reversed by naloxone, suggesting that the effects are not directly related to gabapentin. Instead gabapentin appears to enhance the action of morphine at μ opioid receptors, a pharmacodynamic synergy. This implies that lower doses of morphine combined with gabapentin can be used to produce the same effects when compared to morphine alone.

Other studies have also revealed useful insights into the effects of drug combinations in neuropathic pain. A combination of an opioid (either morphine or methadone) with the N-methyl D-aspartate (NMDA) antagonist ketamine has been given either alone or in combination to rats with a mononeuropathy (caused by ligating the sciatic nerve to produce neuropathic pain). When the neuropathic paw and a normal paw were exposed to pressure testing, synergistic effects were only apparent in the neuropathic paw and not the normal paw. This demonstrates that the opioid–ketamine combination is most effective in the presence of hyperexcitability associated with neuropathic pain, rather than in the context of nociceptive pain.

18.2 **Drug combinations in clinical practice**

The great majority of clinical trials have been conducted with combinations of an opioid and a co-analgesic.

18.2.1 **Opioids with tricyclics**

Tricyclic antidepressants have been studied extensively in the context of neuropathic pain. Amitriptyline has been found to increase plasma morphine through inhibition of hepatic glucuronidation. This potentially allows lower doses of morphine to be given with amitriptyline for the same or better analgesic effect than if morphine is given alone, a pharmacokinetic synergy. Amitriptyline also results in increased expression of leu–enkephalin, a naturally occurring opioid within the central nervous system, which can mimic therapeutic opioid effects. These findings have given rise to the idea that tricyclics are 'opioid sparing'.

A recent clinical trial in patients with post-herpetic neuralgia provides good evidence for using combinations of opioid with tricyclic antidepressants. In this study, patients were entered into a randomized crossover of opioid (morphine or methadone), tricyclic (nortriptyline or desipramine), and placebo. Active drugs reduced pain much more than placebo, as expected. However, patients who experienced good relief with opioid didn't necessarily experience good relief with tricyclics, and vice versa. Although the study did not directly examine the effects of a combination of opioid and tricyclic, it did clearly demonstrate that the active drugs produce analgesia through different mechanisms, suggesting the potential for a pharmacodynamic synergy.

18.2.2 **Opioids with antiepileptics**

Although animal studies have shown a synergistic effect between morphine and gabapentin, clinical evidence in patients has been lacking until recently. A well-designed trial compared the effects of morphine, gabapentin, a combination of both, and placebo in patients with painful diabetic neuropathy or post-herpetic neuralgia. Patients were treated with each arm for five weeks at a time. The final analysis revealed that morphine and gabapentin produced similar analgesic benefits (morphine was slightly better), but the combination resulted in significantly greater analgesia than either drug alone. In fact, the combination consisted of much lower doses of either drug than when used alone. Adverse effects of this combination consisted of constipation, sedation, and dry mouth.

A similar study was also undertaken that added placebo or oxycodone to patients with painful diabetic neuropathy that had reached their maximum tolerated does of gabapentin. The combination group (gabapentin and oxycodone) experienced significantly better pain relief than gabapentin alone.

18.2.3 **Opioids with NMDA antagonists**

Two drugs with activity at the NMDA receptor have been studied in combination with opioids: ketamine and dextromethorphan (see also Chapter 13). When ketamine was given alongside morphine in a small study of cancer patients, whose pain was previously unrelieved by morphine alone, almost all experienced additional analgesic benefit. Adverse effects were frequent, but may reflect the frailty of the patients in the study.

Dextromethorphan has received more attention recently as an NMDA receptor antagonist. It has been combined with morphine in a 1:1 ratio to examine whether it can enhance analgesia or prevent tolerance to chronic opioid administration. Trials lasting around four weeks in a group of patients with mixed cancer and non-cancer pain types (nociceptive, neuropathic) showed that patients receiving the combination needed only half the dose of morphine to achieve good pain control compared to the morphine-only group. Interestingly, a longer trial of three months in non-neuropathic-pain patients failed to show an advantage of the combination over morphine alone. Whether this reflects the fact that any advantage wears off in the longer term, that the amount of dextromethorphan was too low, or that the combination is only effective in the presence of hyperexcitability (see above) is not known.

18.2.4 **Opioids and cholecystokinin antagonists**

Cholecystokinin (CCK) antagonists such as proglumide (see Chapter 12) are known to mediate opioid tolerance in animal models and have been examined in clinical trials. Proglumide has been shown to enhance opioid analgesia, when combined with dihydrocodeine or morphine, in cancer and non-cancer pain. Although these patients did not have exclusive neuropathic pain, this evidence suggests that synergistic effects occur with this combination that may be applicable to neuropathic pain.

18.2.5 **Intrathecal opioids with local anaesthetic or clonidine**

In cases of neuropathic pain that require intrathecal drug delivery (see Chapter 15), combination treatment is often used. Clinical trial evidence clearly supports the addition of clonidine to opioid in this context to enhance analgesia. Local anaesthetic drugs have also been found to enhance opioid analgesia and reduce the development of tolerance. The mechanisms through which these effects occur are not clear.

18.3 **Drug sequencing: stepwise or parallel approaches?**

18.3.1 **A word about NNT and NNH**

The array of drugs that have been examined in neuropathic pain is wide and supported by varying levels of evidence from small case reports to large randomized controlled trials. Condensing this information into a clinically useful management strategy is not easy but is helped by the use of the concepts of number needed to treat (NNT) and number needed to harm (NNH). These respectively refer to the number of patients that need to be treated for one to experience significant pain relief, or significant harm, in comparison with a placebo arm (see also Chapter 11). Significant pain relief is usually taken to mean a reduction in pain score by at least 50%; however, systematic reviews have included trials where 'excellent' or 'good' pain relief occurred (without numerical data), and sometimes 'moderate' pain relief. These different definitions of success will impact on the apparent effectiveness or otherwise of a drug. Also, these analyses may miss important information because they rely on bimodal yes or no criteria.

Recently, a 30% reduction in pain has been demonstrated to be a meaningful benefit for chronic pain patients. Using this less stringent threshold may alter the NNT value of analgesics in future, though evidence to date suggests that using either 30% or 50% threshold gives similar results. No trials have examined improved function as an outcome measure and some analgesics may allow greater activity for the same level of pain. Focusing on pain intensity alone may miss other benefits.

Also important are the confidence intervals (CI) that accompany a derived NNT; wide 95% CI suggest that the NNT has been derived from studies with few patients or that the drug itself has inconsistent effects. Remember also that NNT only tells one side of the story; NNH is also important. Ideally, a drug should have a NNT close to 1 (meaning that almost everyone who is treated experiences significant benefit) and a NNH that is very high (a large majority do not get adverse effects).

It has been argued that earlier studies of treatments in neuropathic pain may have been less able to detect and report adverse events. This would lead to an overestimation of NNH for older antiepileptics and tricyclic antidepressants when compared with more recent studies of co-analgesics, i.e. they appear better tolerated than is the case in clinical practice.

18.3.2 **Benefits and burdens of different approaches**

Stepwise treatment allows a clear relationship between a drug and its beneficial or adverse effects to be established. Patient concordance with medication is likely to be greater and treatment failure allows a drug to be discontinued before a second drug is introduced. This is important in situations where patients are taking medication for other co-morbid conditions and reduces the well-described risks of polypharmacy.

On the other hand, a parallel approach offers the chance of greater pain relief at lower drug doses with potentially fewer adverse effects. Initiating combination therapy may also reduce the time it takes to reach acceptable pain control compared to a stepwise approach. However, combination treatments may result in unpredictable adverse effects either through drug interactions (e.g. some antiepileptics increase plasma levels of tricyclics) or because simultaneous titration of two drugs is more complicated than monotherapy. In addition, successful treatment with a combination approach does not exclude the fact that 1 drug in the combination may be redundant and/or contributing most of the adverse effects.

18.4 **A treatment algorithm**

There are no clinical trials that have tested a sequential approach to treating neuropathic pain. Based on the weight of evidence and experience in clinical practice, suggested approaches to managing neuropathic pain are presented in Table 18.1 (see also Fig. 11.2, Chapter 11). This guidance also reflects UK NICE Clinical Guidelines and a summary published in the BMJ of recent systematic reviews.

18.4.1 **First-line approaches**

A useful first-line approach would be an antidepressant such as amitriptyline or an anti-epileptic such as pregabalin or gabapentin. For diabetic neuropathy there is good evidence that duloxetine can be used as first line treatment. Three studies have compared amitriptyline or nortriptyline directly with gabapentin and have not demonstrated reliably that one is better than the other. However, a combination of a tricyclic antidepressant and gabapentin is superior to either used alone.

Choosing on the basis of adverse effects is probably the best course; for example, amitriptyline would be appropriate for patients who prefer once-daily dosing, have poor sleep, and who are less prone to antimuscarinic effects. Failure on one class (anti-depressant or anti-epileptic) after a four to six-week period of titration would suggest that a trial of the other is indicated. Some experts use low doses of both antidepressants and anti-epileptics as first-line treatment. Additional measures such as TENS, acupuncture, or paracetamol may help.

Table 18.1 Approaches to the management of neuropathic pain

	Monotherapy	Combinations	Additional measures
A. First-line [Referral to specialized pain management service not *necessary*]	Antidepressant, (AD) e.g. amitriptyline or duloxetine Anti-epileptic (AE), e.g. pregabalin or gabapentin	Low-dose AD+AE	Paracetamol TENS Acupuncture
B. Second-line [Referral to specialized pain management service *desirable*]	Capsaicin Lidocaine patch Tizanidine Clonidine Baclofen Alternative antidepressant (e.g. duloxetine if amitriptyline used first line) Opioid: tramadol, morphine, oxycodone (see local protocols)	Opioid with AD or AE	Physiotherapy Occupational therapy
C. Third-line [Referral to specialized pain management service *essential*]	Alternative opioids Ketamine Neuromodulation	Ketamine plus opioid Intrathecal drug delivery	Above plus: Psychological assessment and support

18.4.2 **Second-line approaches**

A second-line step in this sequential approach, after separate trials or combinations of antidepressants and anti-epileptics, might involve a trial of topical measures such as lidocaine patch or capsaicin cream. Other measures such as baclofen or tizanadine may be used. Opioids such as morphine, buprenorphine, tramadol, or oxycodone may be helpful. Morphine and oxycodone have NNT values of around 2.5 and tramadol is recommended by NICE guidance for use in non-specialist settings. It would be important to enter this step after reviewing the clinical diagnosis and ensuring adherence to local protocols (and liaison with local pain management service) for using opioids in non-cancer chronic pain (see Chapter 14). Opioids could replace or be added to either of the drug classes that were used first-line.

18.4.3 **Third-line approaches**

Patients with neuropathic pain that has not improved with initial (and better evidence-based) treatment require additional measures. At this stage, the involvement of a specialized pain management or palliative care service is essential. The use of drugs such as ketamine and alternative opioids, together with neuromodulation, may be undertaken in more specialized facilities that also have access to psychological assessment and support.

18.4.4 **Cancer neuropathic pain**

Treating neuropathic pain in cancer patients as opposed to non-cancer patients may sometimes require a modified approach when prescribing analgesics. The difference is related to the patient rather than pain (see Chapter 9). Cancer patients are more likely to be frail, exhibit a changing pain picture, and have additional renal, hepatic, or cognitive impairment. This means that toxicity may be reached before benefit and therefore the NNT may be higher and NNH may be lower for analgesics in this group. Cancer patients with neuropathic pain or mixed pain types are more likely to have commenced opioid analgesia, and co-analgesic drugs are often combined with opioids to achieve good pain control. A large observational study demonstrated the success of this approach. Early intervention with intrathecal therapy or neurolytic blocks for severe cases is often indicated.

Key references

Dworkin R.H., O'Connor A.B., Backonja M., Farrar J.T., Finnerup N.B., Jensen T.S., Kalso E.A., Loeser J.D., Miaskowski C., Nurmikko T.J., Portenoy R.K., Rice A.S., Stacey B.R., Treede R.D., Turk D.C., Wallace M.S. (2007). Pharmacologic management of neuropathic pain: evidence-based recommendations. *Pain*, **132**(3), 237–51.

Finnerup N.B., Otto M., Jensen T.S. Sindrup S.H. (2007) An evidence-based algorithm for the treatment of neuropathic pain. *Med Gen Med*, **9**(2), 36.

Freynhagen, R., Bennett, M.I. (2009). Diagnosis and management of neuropathic pain. *BMJ*, **339**:b3002. doi:10.1136/bmj.b3002.

Galer B.S., Lee D., Ma T., Nagle B., Schlagheck T.G. (2005). MorphiDex (morphine sulfate/dextromethorphan hydrobromide combination) in the treatment of chronic pain: three multicenter, randomized, double-blind, controlled clinical trials fail to demonstrate enhanced opioid analgesia or reduction in tolerance. *Pain*, **115**(3), 284–95.

Gilron, I., Bailey, J.M., Dongsheng, T., Holden, R.R., Weaver, D.F., Houlden, R.L. (2005). Morphine, gabapentin, or their combination for neuropathic pain. *N Engl J Med*, **352**, 1324–34.

Gilron, I. Bailey, J.M., Tu, D., Holden, R.R., Jackson, A.C., Houlden, R.L. (2009). Nortriptyline and gabapentin, alone and in combination for neuropathic pain: a double-blind, randomised controlled crossover trial. *Lancet*, **374**(9647), 1252–610.

Grond, S., Radbruch, L., Meuser, T., Sabatowski, R., Loick, G., and Lehmann, K.A. (1999). Assessment and treatment of neuropathic cancer pain following WHO guidelines. *Pain*, **79**, 15–20.

Hanna M., O'Brien C., Wilson M.C. (2008). Prolonged-release oxycodone enhances the effects of existing gabapentin therapy in painful diabetic neuropathy patients. *Eur J Pain*, **12**(6), 804–13.

Namaka, M., Gramlich, C.R., Ruhlen, D., Melanson, M., Sutton, I., and Major, J. (2004). A treatment algorithm for neuropathic pain. *Clinical Therapeutics*, **26**, 951–79.

NICE Clinical Guideline (2010). Neuropathic pain: the pharmacological management of neuropathic pain in adults in non-specialist settings. National Institure for Health and Clinical Excellence, London.

Raja, S. N., Haythornthwaite, J.A., Pappagallo, M., Clark, M.R., Travison, T.G., Sabeen, S. *et al.* (2003). Opioids versus antidepressants in postherpetic neuralgia: a randomized, placebo-controlled trial. *Neurology*, **59**, 1015–21.

Chapter 19

Patient perspectives

S. José Closs

19.1 Introduction

19.1.1 Measuring impact on quality of life

Most of our knowledge about neuropathic pain is concerned with its diagnosis and treatment, usually pharmacological. Pain textbooks often provide brief information about the main clinical features of neuropathic pain, but few give a realistic indication of its impact on the lives of patients who suffer from it.

The bizarre nature and unpredictability of this pain may have an enormous negative impact on many aspects of quality of life, including physical, psychological, spiritual, social, and economic aspects of patients' lives. Some aspects have received more attention than others: for example physical and emotional functions can be measured with established scales such as the Brief Pain Inventory. Increasingly, quality of life is being recognized as important and scales such as the Nottingham Health Profile, SF-36, and the EuroQol (EQ-5D) are being used in studies of people with neuropathic pain.

19.1.2 Evidence from patient surveys

There are few large surveys of people with neuropathic pain, but available information suggests that the majority experience severe discomfort due to pain and report that the pain interferes with their general activity, work, sleep, mood, and enjoyment of life (see also Chapter 3). For 126 Swedish patients the most bothersome symptoms resulting from the pain were difficulty sleeping (88%), lack of energy (86%), difficulty in concentrating (76%), and drowsiness (71%) (see Meyer-Rosberg *et al.*). These patients showed poorer physical and social functioning and mental health than the general population. Similarly, 602 Swedish patients showed that neuropathic pain severity was associated with poorer quality-of-life scores (details of these surveys are referenced below).

These tidy epidemiological descriptions of the problems do not communicate what these issues mean at a personal level. This chapter aims to illustrate how some of the key aspects of neuropathic pain impact on the daily lives of individuals. These include quotes from real patients who participated in a qualitative study of the impact of neuropathic pain funded by the British Pain Society (see Appendix 1). The quotes have been selected to illustrate points of major importance to this group.

19.2 Physical and psychological impact

19.2.1 Sleep disturbance and fatigue

Probably the most common problem resulting from neuropathic pain is disrupted sleep. Getting off to sleep, finding a comfortable position, and being woken by pain during the night may all become routine:

> I've not had a full night's sleep in four years...the most I get is three, maybe four hours if I'm lucky.

Considerable physical, emotional, and cognitive efforts are required to live with persistent pain, and sleep loss makes these more difficult. Fatigue may reduce the ability to concentrate due to the distracting nature of pain, making it more difficult to engage with the outside world when actively dealing with the pain.

> ... you can't ignore the whole thing; you can't function, you can't think, you can't concentrate ...

19.2.2 **Emotional and psychological changes**

Some patients reported distressing changes in their mood:

> It [the pain] has affected me where I am bad tempered ... abrupt, snappy, certain times I'm fine, but it doesn't last long ... and then I really feel horrible. And I think why did I do that, and that's what's happening at the moment, this frustration is causing me to change into probably a horrible person.

> ... don't start making out that I'm mentally ill, there's a reason that I'm depressed. ... I've lost all my hobbies. I used to play guitar, ride mountain bikes, all them things have changed — and work's gone, my home's gone. Of course I'm gonna be depressed, I'd be a bloody idiot if I wasn't.

Many expressed concern that their families would become unable or unwilling to live with their negative emotions, and those who recognized the changes in themselves experienced guilt about their effect on their loved ones.

Clearly, those with persistent severe neuropathic pain cope with negative changes in many aspects of their lives. Suicidal ideation was not uncommon among the worst cases:

> I have no life whatsoever you know and I've tried topping myself ... I did try and I laid there just thinking about my grandson and I thought how can you do that, my only grandchild, I love him dearly and he's going to find out that his grandma committed suicide. So I just had glass after glass of salted water and I puked that much ...

19.2.3 **The undesirable side-effects of drugs**

For the most part, medication use was the primary method of attempting to deal with symptoms. This included both prescription and non-prescription drugs, and their effectiveness and side-effects were highly variable:

> I find that if I don't take that [the amitriptyline], the next day I'm like anxious and I think something's going to happen, that fear of something happening, so I have to take them ... I don't know if it's helping me.

> I'm really lethargic, really slow until I get into the afternoon when I feel quite normal, and then I take the tablets again and I go back down.

Increased appetite and the consequent increase in weight as well as a reduced ability to concentrate were additional problems for those taking gabapentin:

> It upsets me—I've got to do something about it. He said to me, 'Well it's a side-effect. Would you rather have the pain?' That's not the point. I'm changing, my body shape, I don't want to look the way I do.

... when I first started taking it I'm thinking I can't concentrate. I couldn't read a book, I still can't read a book really ... I had to make a decision at one point to sort of reduce the gabapentin a little bit and have more pain just to be able to ... A bit more clarity, I won't say brilliant, but a little bit more clarity, yeah.

I feel better now I'm not taking as much. But my concentration, that's something I really suffer with.

19.3 Impact of neuropathic pain on direct social functioning

19.3.1 The impact on family life

Relationships within families became strained, where previously established roles changed. The loss of masculinity or femininity and the inability to fulfill traditional roles such as protecting children or supporting ageing parents produced considerable distress:

Yes, it's a man thing, you've lost all that what men stand for, if you know what I mean. If my daughter gets into trouble, I'm not in a position now to go and sort it out.

... having to ask my dad to come and do it for me, do you know what I mean, and that's just wrong in my eyes. My parents have been there for me all my life and they're at an age now where they should be able to take it easy and rely on their son occasionally to help them out with stuff, and I can't do it for them. They understand, but it doesn't make it any easier from my point of view ...

For some, marital relationships crumbled or broke down altogether:

You know if you're just sort of laid in bed and he puts his hand on my hip to give me a cuddle or anything, I say 'don't touch me' because it's just, it's just I can't even put my own hand there. I certainly don't want anybody else's big hand on me ...'Don't touch me, but you've still got to love me.' [laugh] Strange isn't it? ... And half of the time you're in so much pain you can't be bothered anyway.

I and my husband split up and we'd been married 36 years. We split up because he couldn't stand it any more.

19.3.2 The impact on social activities

Social isolation tended to increase as time went on and friends reduced the frequency of invitations because of the unpredictability of symptoms. Practical difficulties associated with the pain also inhibited social activities:

Yeah, because they ask you out and you're in agony, and nine times out of ten you have to turn round and say 'I'm sorry, I can't make it.' So in the end they think 'what's the point?'

… before the accident, in the summer if it were a nice sunny day you'd just jump in the car and away you went. … You can't do that anymore because you don't know what you're going to be like that day when you wake up …

And when I've got to go shopping … I've got to ask someone, to have someone to lift, and they look at you as if to say 'Are you kidding me?' And, you know, and it's like I can't stand there explaining, I just need the help there and then, and it gets so frustrating.

19.3.3 **Ability to work**

Most patients reported that they attempted to maintain work roles for as long as possible. However, the impact of neuropathic pain symptoms, sleep disruption, and muscle fatigue had severe consequences for some. Those with employers willing to be flexible fared better, but most of those with severe symptoms became resigned to the fact that a return to full-time work was unlikely:

I want to go out to work … One of the pain specialists I went to see over my claims said, 'Oh yeah, he's suitable for work, but he'd have to try and get a job where he could do an hour then clear off for a couple of hours to recover and then come back.' Oh come on, give me a break. Who's going to set you on to do that and pay you for it?

19.4 **Patients with neuropathic pain in the wider society**

19.4.1 **Having their pain reports believed and understood**

A common problem for those with neuropathic pain is being believed and being understood. The invisible nature of pain means that others are unaware of it, unless they have explicitly been told, and even then they may not believe or comprehend the nature and extent of the impact of pain on an individual. This applies to health care professionals, work colleagues, and family and friends. Many patients expressed dissatisfaction with general practitioners (GPs) and pain specialists:

… what's annoying is the person you see is a bog standard GP who's got to make an assessment on something he's got absolute-ly no idea about. I understood what he was saying, there really was nothing they could do, and he said to me, 'Look, people have to cope with pain. Take some tablets and cope.' And at that point I were at my lowest you know, and I said, 'But I feel that I can't live with it.' … If I hadn't have had my family, the way I felt that day I could have quite easily come home and ended it.

Getting friends to understand pain that they couldn't actually see was a difficulty for many:

> You find that people don't believe you a lot of the time, they can't see it so they don't think there's anything the matter with you.

> It's just people's off-the-cuff 'Just get on with it.' ... It's like, what? You wouldn't say that if I came in and I had a bloody leg missing or something. ... You wouldn't react like that if I came in and I had multiple sclerosis or if I had cancer. You don't say to them 'Just bloody get on with it and leave it.'

Not being believed caused sufferers considerable frustration and produced a loss of credibility. Distress also resulted from the notion that psychological problems were the cause of their pain.

> ... everything was so painful ... and you get really a bit depressed with it, and then when you go ... they try and say there's nothing, so they thought it must be psychological and that was the biggest insult for me.

19.4.2 **Their need for accurate information and appropriate support**

Neuropathic pain is difficult to treat successfully, so many sufferers continually sought new treatments and better information (Closs et al. 2007):

> If I take something it's mainly because I've gone to my GP and said I want to try this, because I've been through medical books and I've searched through and thought 'Right, this says it controls muscle spasms and so on. I'll try popping some of them.' And I'll actually go, because it's not nice to go and have someone just say 'Well, go and crack on with it, just get on with it.'

The recent burgeoning of complementary therapies has provided a questionable array of interventions which provide hope for those with neuropathic pain:

> I've tried acupuncture, massage, healing. I've tried everything, because like, you would do. So I have tried quite a lot of alternatives and nothing helps-nothing seems to, it [the pain] seems to have it's own will, it comes and goes.

> I've got self-hypnotism books at home. I'm trying to hypnotize myself and I'm reading and I'm thinking this is just bloody ridiculous, but I still go through the whole book and still sit there for weeks on end. And I couldn't do it.

The lack of consensus between different clinicians was a concern for some, and there was a desire for a single diagnosis and varying amounts of clear information. When doctors disagreed with one another the consequences for the patient were very serious and disempowering:

> I don't know about you but I find that with the different people you see you get so many different opinions.... you're swapping about and for me now I got finished in my job from Dr A in Derby [who] did a medical [for my job] and then ... they said you can't work anymore ... then Dr B at Leeds did the medical for my pension and said, 'Oh you should go to work.' So I lost my job and then I didn't get my pension, so I ended up with nothing, and all on the fact that two people in the same bloody jobs got different opinions.

19.4.3 Potential for improvements in care

It is difficult for health care professionals to help these patients without understanding the genuine unpleasantness of their symptoms and the resulting misery. These experiences are the reason why health care professionals, researchers, and pharmaceutical companies invest so much effort into improving treatments for neuropathic pain. Although the emphasis tends to be on developing new drugs, the content of this chapter suggests that there is scope for improving family and social support, as well as information provision, cognitive therapies, complementary therapies, and perhaps developing other innovative approaches to helping sufferers of chronic neuropathic pain.

Key references

Closs, S.J., Staples, V., Briggs, M., and Bennett, M.I. (2005, unpublished data). *A qualitative study of the experience and impact of neuropathic pain symptoms.* Final report for the British Pain Society, London.

Closs, S.J., Staples, V., Reid I., Bennett, M.I. and Briggs, M. (2007) Managing the symptoms of neuropathic pain: an exploration of patients' experiences. *J Pain and Symptom Man*, **34**(4), 422–33.

McDermott, A.M., Toelle, T.R., Rowbotham, D.J., Schaefer, C.P., and Dukes, E.M. (2006). The burden of neuropathic pain: results from a cross-sectional survey. *Eur J Pain*, **10**, 127–35.

Meyer-Rosberg, K., Burckhardt, C.S., Huizar, K., Kvarnström, A., Nordfors, L., and Kristofferson, A. (2001). A comparison of the SF-36 and Nottingham Health Profile in patients with chronic neuropathic pain. *Eur J Pain*, **5**, 391–403.

Useful links

British Pain Society

British Pain Society
Third Floor Churchill House
35 Red Lion Square
London
WC1R 4SG
UK
www.britishpainsociety.org
info@britishpainsociety.org

BPS website contains position statement on 'The use of drugs beyond licence in palliative care and pain management' plus accompanying patient information leaflet. BPS has also published guidelines on opioids in persistent non-cancer pain and spinal cord stimulation.

Pain Relief Foundation

Pain Relief Foundation
Clinical Sciences Centre
University Hospital Aintree
Lower Lane
Liverpool
L9 7AL
UK
www.painrelieffoundation.org.uk

The Neuropathy Trust

The Neuropathy Trust
PO Box 26
Nantwich
Cheshire
CW5 5FP
UK
www.neurocentre.com
admin@neurocentre.com

Martindale Pharma Ltd

Martindale Pharmaceuticals Ltd
Bampton Road
Harold Hill
Romford
Essex

RM3 8UG
UK
Customer Services
Tel: 0800 0287933
Fax: 0800 0287944
www.martindalepharma.co.uk

Palliative Care Formulary on-line

www.palliativedrugs.com

International Association for the Study of Pain (IASP)

IASP
111 Queen Anne Avenue N
Suite 501
Seattle
WA 98109-4955
USA
www.iasp-pain.org

American Pain Society

American Pain Society
4700 W Lake Avenue
Glenview
IL 60025
USA
www.ampainsoc.org
info@ampainsoc.org
secretary@painrelieffoundation.org.uk

The Neuropathy Association

The Neuropathy Association
60 E 42nd Street
Suite 942
New York
NY 10165
USA
www.neuropathy.org

Australian Pain Society

Suite 1 Ground floor
26 Ridge St
North Sydney NSW 2060
Australia
www.apsoc.org.au

Appendix 2

Neuropathic pain descriptor scales

Leeds Assessment of Neuropathic Symptoms and Signs (LANSS)

Bennett, M. (2001). The LANSS pain scale: the Leeds Assessment of Neuropathic Symptoms and Signs. *Pain*, **92**, 147–57.

THE LANSS PAIN SCALE
Leeds Assessment of Neuropathic Symptoms and Signs

NAME _____ DATE _____

This pain scale can help to determine whether the nerves that are carrying your pain signals are working normally or not. It is important to find this out in case different treatments are needed to control your pain.

A. PAIN QUESTIONNAIRE

Think about <u>how your pain has felt over the last week</u>.

Please say whether any of the descriptions match your pain exactly.

1. **Does your pain feel like strange, unpleasant sensations in your skin? Words like 'pricking', 'tingling', 'pins and needles' might describe these sensations.**

   a) NO – My pain doesn't really feel like this................................. (0)

   b) YES – I get these sensations quite a lot.. (5)

2. **Does your pain make the skin in the painful area look different from normal? Words like 'mottled' or 'looking more red or pink' might describe the appearance.**

   a) NO – My pain doesn't affect the colour of my skin..................... (0)

   b) YES – I've noticed that the pain does make my skin look different from normal.... (5)

3. **Does your pain make the affected skin abnormally sensitive to touch? Getting unpleasant sensations when lightly stroking the skin, or getting pain when wearing tight clothes might describe the abnormal sensitivity.**

   a) NO – My pain doesn't make my skin abnormally sensitive in that area.......... (0)

   b) YES – My skin seems abnormally sensitive to touch in that area.................... (3)

4. **Does your pain come on suddenly and in bursts for no apparent reason when you're still? Words like 'electric shocks', 'jumping', and 'bursting' describe these sensations.**

   a) NO – My pain doesn't really feel like this.. (0)

   b) YES – I get these sensations quite a lot... (2)

5. **Does your pain feel as if the skin temperature in the painful area has changed abnormally? Words like 'hot' and 'burning' describe these sensations.**

   a) NO – I don't really get these sensations.. (0)

   b) YES – I get these sensations quite a lot.. (1)

B. SENSORY TESTING

Skin sensitivity can be examined by comparing the painful area with a contralateral or adjacent non-painful area for the presence of allodynia and an altered pinprick threshold (PPT).

1. ALLODYNIA

Examine the response to lightly stroking cotton wool across the non-painful area and then the painful area. If normal sensations are experienced in the non-painful site, but pain or unpleasant sensations (tingling, nausea) are experienced in the painful area when stroking, allodynia is present.

   a) NO, normal sensation in both areas... (0)

   b) YES, allodynia in painful area only... (5)

2. ALTERED PINPRICK THRESHOLD

Determine the pinprick threshold by comparing the response to a 23-gauge (blue) needle mounted inside a 2ml syringe barrel placed gently on to the skin in non-painful and then painful areas.

If a sharp pinprick is felt in the non-painful area, but a different sensation is experienced in the painful area, e.g. none/blunt only (raised PPT) or a very painful sensation (lowered PPT), an altered PPT is present.

If a pinprick is not felt in either area, mount the syringe onto the needle to increase the weight and repeat.

   a) NO, equal sensation in both areas... (0)

   b) YES, altered PPT in painful area... (3)

....

192

SCORING:

Add values in parentheses for sensory description and examination findings to obtain overall score.

TOTAL SCORE (maximum 24) ....

If score <12, neuropathic mechanisms are **unlikely** to be contributing to the patient's pain.

If score ≥12, neuropathic mechanisms are **likely** to be contributing to the patient's pain.

Self-report LANSS (S-LANSS)

Bennett, M.I., Smith, B.H., Torrance, N., Potter, J. (2005). The S-LANSS score for identifying pain of predominantly neuropathic origin: validation for use in clinic and postal research. *J Pain*, **6**, 149–58.

THE S-LANSS PAIN SCORE

Leeds Assessment of Neuropathic Symptoms and Signs (self-complete)

NAME _____   DATE _____

- This questionnaire can tell us about the type of pain that you may be experiencing. This can help in deciding how best to treat it.
- Please draw on the diagram below where you feel your pain. If you have pain in more than one area, **only shade in the one main area where your worst pain is.**

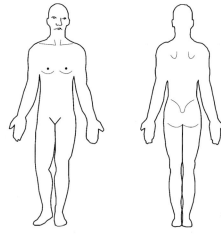

- On the scale below, please indicate how bad your pain (that you have shown on the above diagram) has been in the last week where:

  '0' means no pain and '10' means pain as severe as it could be.

NONE   0   1   2   3   4   5   6   7   8   9   10   **SEVERE PAIN**

- On the other side of the page are 7 questions about your pain (the one in the diagram).
- Think about how your pain that you showed in the diagram has felt **over the last week.** Put a tick against the descriptions that best match your pain. These descriptions may, or may not, match your pain, no matter how severe it feels.
- Only circle the responses that describe your pain. **Please turn over.**

S-LANSS

1. In the area where you have pain, do you also have 'pins and needles', tingling, or prickling sensations?

   a) NO – I don't get these sensations (0)

   b) YES – I get these sensations often (5)

2. Does the painful area change colour (perhaps looks mottled or more red) when the pain is particularly bad?

   a) NO – The pain does not affect the colour of my skin (0)

   b) YES – I have noticed that the pain does make my skin look different from normal (5)

3. Does your pain make the affected skin abnormally sensitive to touch? Getting unpleasant sensations or pain when lightly stroking the skin might describe this.

   a) NO – The pain does not make my skin in that area abnormally sensitive to touch (0)

   b) YES – My skin in that area is particularly sensitive to touch (3)

4. Does your pain come on suddenly and in bursts for no apparent reason when you are completely still? Words like 'electric shocks', 'jumping', and 'bursting' might describe this.

   a) NO – My pain doesn't really feel like this (0)

   b) YES – I get these sensations often (2)

5. In the area where you have pain, does your skin feel unusually hot like a burning pain?

   a) NO – I don't have burning pain (0)

   b) YES – I get burning pain often (1)

6. Gently <u>rub</u> the painful area with your index finger and then rub a non-painful area (for example, an area of skin further away or on the opposite side from the painful area). How does this rubbing feel in the painful area?

   a) The painful area feels no different from the non-painful area (0)

   b) I feel discomfort, like pins and needles, tingling, or burning in the painful area that is different from the non-painful area (5)

7. Gently <u>press</u> on the painful area with your fingertip then gently press in the same way onto a non-painful area (the same non-painful area that you chose in the last question). How does this feel in the painful area?

   a) The painful area does not feel different from the non-painful area (0)

   b) I feel numbness or tenderness in the painful area that is different from the non-painful area (3)

Scoring: a score of 12 or more suggests pain of predominantly neuropathic origin.

Neuropathic Pain Scale (NPS)

Galer, B.S. and Jensen, M.P. (1997). Development and preliminary validation of a pain measure specific to neuropathic pain: the Neuropathic Pain Scale. *Neurology*, **48**, 332–8.

The NPS is distributed through the MAPI website—www.mapi-research.fr/. The NPS is free to use in clinical practice but a fee is payable to use in funded research projects.

Neuropathic Pain Symptom Inventory (NPSI)

Bouhassira, D., Attal, N., Fermanian, J., Alchaar, H., Gautron, M., Masquelier, E., *et al.* (2004). Development and validation of the Neuropathic Pain Symptom Inventory. *Pain*, **108**, 248–57.

Douleur Neuropathique 4 (DN4)

Bouhassira, D., Attal, N., Alchaar, H., Boureau, F., Brochet, B.,Bruxelle, J., *et al.* (2005). Comparison of pain syndromes associated with nervous or somatic lesions and development of a new neuropathic pain diagnostic questionnaire (DN4). *Pain*, **114**, 29–36.

Neuropathic Pain Questionnaire (NPQ)

Krause, S.J. and Backonja, M.M. (2003). Development of a neuropathic pain questionnaire. *Clin. J. Pain*, **19**, 306–14.

painDETECT

Freynhagen R, Baron R, Gockel U, Tolle TR. painDETECT (2006) a new screening questionnaire to identify neuropathic components in patients with back pain. *Curr Med Res Opin*, **22**(10), 1911–20.

Index

Please note that page references relating to non-textual content such as Boxes, Figures or Tables are in *italic* print.

D

E

F

G

H

I